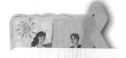

Bladder Cancer

D0863493

EDITED BY

Mark L. Gonzalgo, MD, PhD

Former Associate Professor of Urology,
The James Buchanan Brady Urological Institute
The Johns Hopkins Medical Institutions
Baltimore, Maryland

Associate Professor of Urology,
Department of Urology
Stanford University School of Medicine
Stanford, California

SERIES EDITORS

Lillie D. Shockney, RN, BS, MAS

University Distinguished Service Assistant Professor of Breast Cancer; Administrative Director of Breast
Cancer; Assistant Professor, Department of Surgery; Assistant Professor, Department of Obstetrics and
Gynecology, Johns Hopkins School of Medicine; Assistant Professor, Johns Hopkins School of Nursing

Gary R. Shapiro, MD

Chairman, Department of Oncology
Johns Hopkins Bayview Medical Center
Director, Johns Hopkins Geriatric Oncology Program
The Sidney Kimmel Comprehensive Cancer Center at Johns Hopkins

World Headquarters

Jones and Bartlett Publishers	Jones and Bartlett Publishers	Jones and Bartlett Publishers
40 Tall Pine Drive	Canada	International
Sudbury, MA 01776	6339 Ormindale Way	Barb House, Barb Mews
978-443-5000	Mississauga, Ontario L5V 1J2	London W6 7PA
info@jbpub.com	Canada	United Kingdom
www.jbpub.com		

Jones and Bartlett's books and products are available through most bookstores and online booksellers. To contact Jones and Bartlett Publishers directly, call 800-832-0034, fax 978-443-8000, or visit our website at www.jbpub.com.

Substantial discounts on bulk quantities of Jones and Bartlett's publications are available to corporations, professional associations, and other qualified organizations. For details and specific discount information, contact the special sales department at Jones and Bartlett via the above contact information or send an email to specialsales@jbpub.com.

The author, editors, and publisher have made every effort to provide accurate information. However, they are not responsible for errors, omissions, or for any outcomes related to the use of the contents of this book and take no responsibility for the use of the products and procedures described. Treatments and side effects described in this book may not be applicable to all people; likewise, some people may require a dose or experience a side effect that is not described herein. Drugs and medical devices are discussed that may have limited availability controlled by the Food and Drug Administration (FDA) for use only in a research study or clinical trial. Research, clinical practice, and government regulations often change the accepted standard in this field. When consideration is being given to use of any drug in the clinical setting, the healthcare provider or reader is responsible for determining FDA status of the drug, reading the package insert, and reviewing prescribing information for the most up-to-date recommendations on dose, precautions, and contraindications, and determining the appropriate usage for the product. This is especially important in the case of drugs that are new or seldom used.

Production Credits
Executive Publisher: Christopher Davis
Senior Editorial Assistant: Jessica Acox
Editorial Assistant: Sara Cameron
Associate Production Editor: Katie Spiegel
Senior Marketing Manager: Barb Bartoszek
V.P., Manufacturing and Inventory Control: Therese Connell
Composition: Appingo Publishing Services
Cover Design: Kristin E. Parker
Cover Image: © ImageZoo/age fotostock
Printing and Binding: Malloy, Inc.
Cover Printing: Malloy, Inc.

Library of Congress Cataloging-in-Publication Data

Gonzalgo, Mark L.
  Johns Hopkins patients' guide to bladder cancer / Mark L. Gonzalgo.
    p. cm.
  Includes index.
  ISBN 978-0-7637-7424-0
  1. Bladder cancer—Popular works. I. Title. II. Title: Guide to bladder cancer.
  RC280.B5G66 2011
  616.99'462—dc22

                                                      2009040804

6048

Printed in the United States of America

13 12 11 10 09   10 9 8 7 6 5 4 3 2 1

Contents

Preface

Receiving a diagnosis of bladder cancer is overwhelming. Bladder cancer is a complex disease that can range from a nonaggressive form to a much more serious problem. Depending on the type of bladder cancer that may affect you or your loved one, there are many treatment options. Trying to determine your next steps following the diagnosis is challenging.

Remember that you are not alone. Over 70,000 people were diagnosed with bladder cancer in the United States in 2009. Empowering yourself with information is an important step to making informed decisions and finding out which treatment option is best for you.

This book is part of a series of Johns Hopkins Cancer Patient Guides designed to educate newly diagnosed patients about their cancer diagnosis and the treatment that may lie ahead. The information provided will guide patients and their support teams of family and friends from the time cancer is confirmed to the completion of treatment.

Don't feel the need to read the entire book at once. It is intended for you to read at your leisure and when you feel ready for additional information. Resource information, including access to Johns Hopkins oncology specialists, is also contained within these pages.

Mark L. Gonzalgo, MD, PhD
Former Associate Professor of Urology,
The James Buchanan Brady Urological Institute
The Johns Hopkins Medical Institutions
Baltimore, Maryland

Associate Professor of Urology,
Department of Urology
Stanford University School of Medicine
Stanford, California

DEDICATION

This book is dedicated to all patients with bladder cancer who we have had the privilege of caring for and treating at Johns Hopkins. I hope that the information contained within these pages helps to make the decision-making process regarding your treatment plan less confusing. We are constantly pursuing better ways to diagnose and treat this complex disease. It is my hope that one day we will be able to find a cure for bladder cancer.

Mark L. Gonzalgo

Contributors

Mark W. Ball
Medical Student,
The Johns Hopkins University School of Medicine
Baltimore, Maryland

Kristen A. Burns, CRNP
Adult Urology Nurse Practitioner,
The James Buchanan Brady Urological Institute
The Johns Hopkins University School of Medicine
Baltimore, Maryland

Charles G. Drake, MD, PhD
Associate Professor of Oncology, Immunology
    and Urology,
Johns Hopkins Kimmel Cancer Center
Baltimore, Maryland

Thomas J. Guzzo, MD
Assistant Professor of Urology,
Division of Urology, Department of Surgery
University of Pennsylvania School of Medicine
Philadelphia, Pennsylvania

Brian McNeil, MD
Fellow in Urologic Oncology,
Department of Urology
Memorial Sloan-Kettering Cancer Center
New York, New York

Phillip Pierorazio, MD
Resident in Urology,
The James Buchanan Brady Urological Institute
The Johns Hopkins University School of Medicine
Baltimore, Maryland

Wilmer B. Roberts, MD, PhD
Chief Resident in Urology,
The James Buchanan Brady Urological Institute
The Johns Hopkins University School of Medicine
Baltimore, Maryland

Charlene Rogers, MSN, RN
Research/Clinical Nurse Coordinator,
The James Buchanan Brady Urological Institute
The Johns Hopkins University School of Medicine
Baltimore, Maryland

Mark P. Schoenberg, MD
Professor of Urology,
The James Buchanan Brady Urological Institute
The Johns Hopkins University School of Medicine
Baltimore, Maryland

Gary R. Shapiro, MD
Chairman, Department of Oncology,
Johns Hopkins Bayview Medical Center
Director, Johns Hopkins Geriatric Oncology Program
Baltimore, Maryland

Joanne Walker, MS, RN, CWOCN
Ostomy Nurse Specialist,
The Johns Hopkins Hospital
Baltimore, Maryland

Introduction

How to Use This Book to Your Benefit

You will receive a great deal of information from your healthcare team. You will also probably seek out some information on the Internet or in bookstores. No doubt friends and family members, meaning well, will probably offer you advice on what to do and when to do it, and will try to steer you in certain directions. Relax. Yes, you have heard words you wish you had never heard said about you, that you have bladder cancer. Despite that shocking phrase, you have time to make good decisions and to empower yourself with accurate information so that you can participate in the decision making about your care and treatment.

This book is designed to be a how-to guide that will take you through the maze of treatment options and sometimes complicated schedules, and will help you put together a plan of action so that you become a bladder cancer survivor.

This book is broken down into chapters and includes an index as well as credible resources listed for your further review and education. By empowering yourself with understandable information, we hope you will be comfortable participating in the decision making about your treatment.

Let's begin now with understanding what has happened and what the steps are to get you well again.

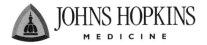
JOHNS HOPKINS
MEDICINE

FIRST STEPS—
I'VE BEEN DIAGNOSED
WITH BLADDER CANCER

BRIAN MCNEIL, MD

You've recently been told you may have bladder cancer. You may have had a CT scan (also called a CAT scan) or MRI for some other reason or recently undergone cystoscopy, a procedure performed by a urologist in which your bladder is examined with a small scope. You may be surprised by the diagnosis because you may not have had any symptoms other than blood in your urine or difficulties urinating. You might be asking yourself, "How is this possible?" or "Why is this happening to me?" Bladder cancer is more common than you think, and in this book we discuss what a diagnosis of bladder cancer means for you and what can be done about it. In this chapter we focus on the first steps one should take after being diagnosed with bladder cancer. Before moving on, I'll give you a bit of background information about the urinary system and bladder cancer.

BACKGROUND INFORMATION

The urinary system (**Figure 1-1**) is very important and has a pretty tough job to do in everyone's body. It filters your blood and produces waste products in the form of urine. More importantly, it allows you to store urine until it is convenient to urinate. Just think, if we couldn't store urine, then we would constantly leak waste products. This would make life very difficult and get in the way of things we do during the course of a normal day. The human urinary system is made up of the kidneys, ureters, bladder, and urethra. Men have a prostate gland in addition to the previously mentioned components.

KIDNEYS

Your kidneys are two bean-shaped organs that reside in the rear of your abdomen, just under the diaphragm on the left and below the liver on your right side. The kidneys filter blood and produce urine. They are extremely important to life and work extremely hard to filter waste from your bloodstream. Just imagine, the kidneys filter approximately 20 percent of your blood each minute. Although most people have two kidneys, some individuals have one and do just fine. The kidneys function independently, and when one is not working as well, the other compensates and filters more blood. In addition to filtering blood and producing urine, your kidneys help to regulate your blood pressure. They produce special hormones and control the salt and water balance in your body. Normally, the kidneys do not release blood cells into urine. This is why it's important to be evaluated by a doctor if you have blood in your urine.

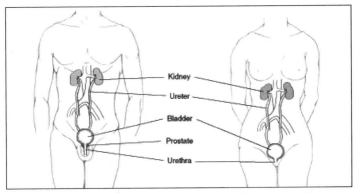

Figure 1-1   Genitourinary system in the male (left) and female (right). The kidneys produce urine that travels down the ureter and into the bladder where it is store before exiting the body via the urethra. The urethra in males is longer than in females and passes through the prostate before exiting the body.

URETERS

After urine is formed by the kidneys, special nerves and muscles in the renal pelvis propel urine downward into the ureters. The ureters are small tubes, very much like the renal pelvis, that allow passage of urine from the kidneys down to the bladder. They function as drainage pipes for the kidney. The ureters have nerves and layers of muscle that propel urine to the bladder. There is so much that your body does that you may not realize. Like the renal pelvis, the ureters are also lined with transitional cells serving as a continuation of the urothelium.

BLADDER

The ureters connect to the bladder, which is a muscular, balloon-like structure in the pelvis. The bladder functions as the storage unit of the urinary system. It can hold upward of 500–600 mL (2 cups) of urine. The bladder is very thick and elastic with multiple layers (**Figure 1-2**): an inner

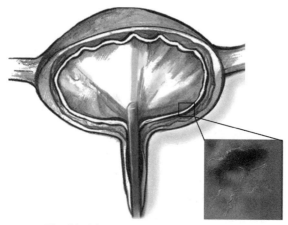

Figure 1-2   The bladder is comprised of multiple tissue layers that are important to understand when talking about your pathology report. A urologist typically will make a diagnosis of bladder cancer using a cytoscope to look into your bladder (shown here).

layer made up of transitional cells forming the urothelium; under this lies a thin layer (the lamina propria), with blood vessels supplying the bladder; and finally a thick muscular layer that contracts to empty your bladder. There is a layer of fat surrounding the muscular layer.

The bladder expands in relation to the amount of fluid inside of it. Bladder contraction is under complex control by your central nervous system. When your bladder contracts during urination, urine passes though the urethra before leaving your body.

URETHRA

The urethra is a hollow tube lined with transitional cells at its beginning that connects the bladder to the outside world. The structure of the urethra is different in men and women. The urethra is short in women and is much longer in men due to the presence of the penis. The cells lining the urethra change along its length. The inner cells, closest to the bladder, are transitional cells, whereas the cells closest to the outside of the body are squamous cells resembling skin. Although the urethra has different lengths in men and women, it functions the same. In men, the urethra passes through the prostate gland near the bladder.

PROSTATE

The prostate, a walnut-sized organ that lies at the base of the bladder in men, plays a role in male fertility. Along with the seminal vesicles, the prostate gland produces fluid that helps sperm after ejaculation. Although the urethra passes through the prostate, the gland itself does not add much, if anything, to the volume of urine that reaches the bladder. As the urethra passes through the prostate, it is lined by transitional cells comprising the urothelium. Therefore, things that affect the urothelium can affect the prostate as well. This is very important when it comes to staging bladder cancer.

WHAT YOU SHOULD KNOW BEFORE YOUR FIRST VISIT

WHAT IS CANCER?

Cancer is defined as a group of diseases characterized by uncontrolled growth and spread of abnormal cells. Cells are the small building blocks of our body and most other living organisms. If the spread of these abnormal cells is not controlled, it can result in organ dysfunction and death. There are several cancers, each affecting various portions of the body. Cancer can be caused by external factors like cigarette smoking, exposure to certain chemicals, radiation, or infectious organisms. Internal factors that can lead to cancer include inherited mutations, hormones, and conditions affecting your immune system. Mutations are permanent changes in your hereditary material, and hormones are products of certain cells in our body that influence the function of other cells.

Although scientists have been able to uncover the cause of some cancers, there is still a great deal to be learned. One may go through his or her entire life without exposure to any of the previously mentioned factors and develop cancer. Men have a higher risk of developing cancer, with a slightly less than 1 in 2 lifetime risk in the United States compared with 1 in 3 for women. Although cancer is more common than you may think, doctors have figured out new ways to diagnose and treat cancer. By no means is cancer a death sentence; it can be managed and a lot of people diagnosed go on to live healthy and productive lives for many years after treatment.

BLADDER CANCER EPIDEMIOLOGY

Epidemiology is essentially the study of factors affecting the health and illness of populations. Before moving on with our discussion about bladder cancer, it's important to gain perspective on how many people live with bladder cancer.

There are over 1 million people throughout the world living with bladder cancer. Bladder cancer is the seventh or ninth most common cancer, depending on where you live. Most individuals with bladder cancer live in industrialized countries and geographical areas where infection with the parasite *Schistosoma haematobium* is common. In the United States bladder cancer is the fourth most common cancer in men and the ninth most frequently diagnosed cancer in women. The male-to-female ratio is 3 to 1. Two-thirds of cases are diagnosed in people over age 60, but it can occur very early in life. Two times as many whites will be diagnosed with bladder cancer compared with African Americans. The reasons for this are unclear.

WHAT CAUSES BLADDER CANCER?

Ludwig Rehn, a German surgeon during the 19th century, is credited with the first explanation of one of the root causes of bladder cancer. He established a link between exposure to chemicals used in the production of colored textiles and the development of bladder cancer in factory workers. Although his discovery was not initially accepted, bladder cancer was soon recognized as an occupational cancer in factory workers. This may help explain the higher incidence of bladder cancer in industrialized nations.

Exposure to a number of chemicals has been associated with the development of bladder cancer. These include aniline dyes and other members of the aromatic amine family. People who work in occupations where exposure to these chemicals is common include textile workers, dye workers, rubber workers, painters, and even hairdressers. Please see **Table 1-1** for a list of occupations associated with an increased risk of developing bladder cancer.

Smoking is the most common cause of bladder cancer today. It increases your risk of developing bladder cancer 2- to 4-fold compared with people who don't smoke. The risk of bladder cancer increases with the frequency and duration of smoking. For example, someone who smokes one pack a day for 20 years has a higher risk of bladder cancer than someone who smokes a few cigarettes on weekends. When you stop smoking you can slowly decrease the risk of bladder cancer, over the course of 20–30 years. If you currently smoke, it would be best to stop smoking

Table 1-1   Occupations at Increased Risk of Developing
Bladder Cancer

- Textile workers
- Tire and rubber workers
- Bootblacks
- Truck drivers
- Dye workers
- Leather workers
- Painters
- Hairdressers who work with dyes
- Drill press operators
- Petroleum workers
- Dry cleaners
- Chemical workers
- Aluminum workers

immediately. Some scientists believe this may help improve your outcome from treatment. If you smoke a pipe or cigar, you may also have an increased risk for developing bladder cancer, but cigarettes are the main culprit behind bladder cancer today.

Chronic inflammation of your bladder may also place you at an increased risk of developing a specific type of bladder cancer called squamous cell carcinoma. Inflammation occurs when one has an untreated urinary tract infection, bladder stones, an indwelling bladder catheter, or an infection with a parasite called *Schistosoma haematobium*. Paraplegics or quadriplegics who require a catheter to drain their bladders and those who live in areas where *S. haematobium* is common are at greatest risk.

Saridon (phenacetin) and Cytoxan (cyclophosphamide) are two other substances that can increase your risk of bladder cancer. Phenacetin is a pain medicine that is no longer used that was previously shown to be associated with bladder cancer. Cytoxan is a drug used for chemotherapy that has been associated with bladder cancer. This may sound puzzling as you wonder, "how does one drug used to treat cancer cause another cancer?" Cytoxan itself is not the problem. Most medications are broken down by our bodies into components before being eliminated in our stool or urine. One of the byproducts of cyclophosphamide, called acrolein, can irritate the wall of your bladder, causing a lot of blood in your urine. Over time, this can increase the risk of developing bladder cancer.

A history of radiation therapy for a pelvic cancer may increase your risk of bladder cancer. Radiation has a role in the treatment of prostate, cervical, and ovarian cancers. Although the radiation is focused on the involved organ, the bladder and other surrounding structures also absorb radiation that sometimes damages the urothelium and leads to cancer.

Much attention has been paid to the influence of diet on cancer risk and treatment. Thus far, some scientists have suggested that vegetables, fresh fruits, and some fermented milk products appear to decrease one's risk of developing bladder cancer. A few foods thought to increase the risk of developing bladder cancer are foods rich in animal fat, those containing a lot of cholesterol, fried foods, and processed meat with various additives. We are not sure of the exact influence of diet on bladder cancer at this point in time. Scientists around the world are working on uncovering potential links between diet and bladder cancer.

ARE THERE VARIOUS TYPES OF BLADDER CANCER?

As with other cancers that affect different body parts, there are multiple types of bladder cancer. To better understand them, let's separate bladder cancer into two different groups: primary tumors that originate in the bladder and secondary tumors that spread to the bladder from other places.

Primary bladder cancers form within the bladder. Over 90 percent of primary bladder cancers in the United States are of the urothelial or transitional subtype. These form along the inner lining of the bladder. The second most common type of primary bladder cancer in the United States is squamous cell carcinoma, making up approximately 5 percent of all cancers diagnosed. These are often diagnosed in individuals whose bladder has been chronically irritated by an infection, stones, or an indwelling catheter. The third most common subtype of bladder cancer in the United States is adenocarcinoma, accounting for approximately 2 percent of all diagnosed cases. These typically form near the dome of the bladder. There are other types of primary bladder cancer, but these are very rare. If necessary, your urologist will speak to you about these rare types.

Secondary cancers form somewhere else in the body and spread to the bladder. Other tumors can get to the bladder by using the bloodstream, your lymphatic system, or directly from an organ close to the bladder. Other cancers that spread to the bladder, in order of decreasing frequency, are melanoma, colon cancer, prostate cancer, lung cancer, and breast cancer.

Now that we've discussed some of the basics concerning bladder cancer, let's examine how you should go about choosing a medical team to treat your cancer.

HOW TO SELECT YOUR ONCOLOGY TEAM
AND BLADDER CANCER CENTER

You want your team to be knowledgeable and experienced in the care of patients with bladder cancer. Don't rely on self-promoting advertisements on television as your way to select a facility and doctor. While you may seek out a comprehensive cancer center (look for one accredited by American College of Surgeons or National Cancer Institute), the important thing is that you select a facility that has bladder cancer specialists. These include urologists that specialize in cancer surgeries (not general urologists or surgeons who rarely perform cancer-related surgery), medical oncologists who specialize in bladder cancer, radiation oncologists, urologic pathologists, radiologists, genetics counselors, oncology nurses, and psychosocial support staff for cancer patients. It's a highly specialized group. Your doctors and their staffs can be some of your best resources.

When you see your urologist, ask questions:

- How many bladder cancer surgeries do you do a year?

- What other types of surgeries do you do, and therefore how much time do you spend doing bladder cancer treatment?

- How often do your patients require additional treatment such as chemotherapy or radiation after surgery?

- What is the best urinary diversion option for me (ileal conduit, catheterizable stoma, neobladder) and why?

- Are you board certified? In what specialty?

- How long have you been in practice?

- Do you regularly attend urologic cancer tumor boards to present cases for team discussion?

- Do you work with a multidisciplinary team of oncologists who also specialize in bladder cancer so that continuity of care can be maintained?

- What is your philosophy on educating patients about their treatment options?

These are all questions that you have the right to have answered before deciding that this doctor is to be your urologic oncology surgeon. If he or she hesitates before answering, consider that this person may not be the doctor you want to have performing your surgery.

WHAT SHOULD YOU DO BEFORE YOUR FIRST APPOINTMENT?

Before visiting your bladder cancer specialist for the first time, you should gather all of your medical records. It is important to obtain copies of your biopsy and cytology reports, radiology studies, operative reports and any other test reports related to your diagnosis of bladder cancer. In addition to written reports, you should request your actual pathology slides for review by the urological pathologist who works with your urologist. It is also important to obtain actual copies of any radiological exams performed. Often, you can obtain a CD with your exams on it or actual films.

WHAT IS A BIOPSY?

A biopsy is a small piece of tissue obtained during cystoscopy when a urologist looks inside of your bladder. This tissue sample is then sent to the laboratory and looked at under a microscope by a pathologist. Although there are standards that all pathologists follow, there can be small differences that can be seen by a trained eye. This is why it's important to obtain actual slides and not just the report.

In addition to biopsies, pathologists often look at urine specimens or bladder washings for the presence of abnormal cells. It's important to bring this report to your first appointment as well.

RADIOLOGICAL STUDIES

Before your referral to a bladder cancer specialist, your primary care provider or urologist may order one of a few radiology exams to help evaluate the extent of cancer. We'll briefly discuss those tests commonly ordered during the workup of someone with bladder cancer. These tests help determine someone's cancer stage. Again, it is very important to obtain copies of your images (the actual films or CDs) along with reports.

An ultrasound is a noninvasive test used to evaluate the kidneys and bladder. Ultrasounds are painless and don't have any associated side effects. Ultrasounds are performed by either a radiologist or radiology technician and take approximately 30 minutes to complete. An ultrasound allows doctors to image your kidneys to determine whether or not they are normal in size. An ultrasound can also determine if one of your kidneys is not draining properly, which can occur with bladder cancer. Although images of your bladder can be obtained, an ultrasound cannot rule out evidence of cancer. Ultrasound was a primary test used in the past to evaluate patients with bladder cancer; however, we now have better tests that allow us to image your entire urinary tract in greater detail. Ultrasound pros include its noninvasiveness and lack of radiation, whereas its cons remain its lack of fine details and the fact that some very small tumors can be missed.

An intravenous pyelogram, or IVP, is a test used to define the anatomy of your urinary tract using intravenous dye and an x-ray machine. Doctors order this test to determine whether or not there are any blockages or tumors in the renal pelvis, ureter, or bladder. Often, patients are asked to have a light meal the night before an IVP and to skip breakfast the morning of the exam. You may be given instructions to perform a bowel prep using magnesium citrate, a laxative available in your local pharmacy or supermarket. This clears out your small intestine and colon as these may interfere with visualization of your urinary tract. If you have diabetes and are using Glucophage (metformin), you may need to stop these medications several days in advance. This should be coordinated by your urologist and primary care physician.

IVPs can take an hour to perform because images are taken of your abdomen at various time points. You may feel a warm sensation, become nauseated, or have a metallic taste in your mouth when the dye is injected.

There are several reasons why you should *not* have an IVP performed, and these will be explained by your doctor. If you have an allergy to IV dye, you could have a potentially severe allergic reaction. In some cases, steroids are given to prevent this from occurring. Either way, this is something that must be discussed with your doctor before the exam. If you have abnormal kidney function, another test will most likely be performed instead of an IVP. This is because the IV dye can worsen your kidney function. If you are pregnant, another test will be performed because of the potentially small risk that the radiation from the x-ray machine poses to the developing fetus. If you have asthma, multiple myeloma, sickle cell disease, pheochromocytoma, or a tumor of your adrenal gland, your physician may order another test because you may also be at greater risk of complications from the exam.

IVP pros include its ability to assess how well your kidneys are working and the images that it can obtain of your renal pelvis and ureter. Its cons include x-ray radiation exposure in addition to the risks of an allergic reaction to IV contrast and potential worsening of borderline kidney function. IVPs are still ordered to evaluate people with blood in their urine or a diagnosis of bladder cancer, but it is slowly being replaced by other, more accurate imaging modalities including CT scan and MRI.

A CT, or CAT scan, is a computed tomographic scan that obtains accurate, detailed images of the body and its contents. It allows radiologists to look at detailed images of all your internal organs, including your heart, lungs, liver, brain, kidneys, and bladder, in addition to soft tissues like lymph nodes. CT scans are performed in radiology departments by radiologists with the assistance of nurses and technicians. The actual exam may only last 15 minutes, but you may be in the radiology area for an hour. As with the preparation for an IVP, you will be asked to eat a light dinner the night before, and some doctors prefer bowel preparation with a laxative the day before. You should not eat anything in the 8 hours before your scheduled appointment. Those with diabetes using Glucophage must stop taking these medications several days before the scan if IV dye will be used and will not be able to resume use of these medications for 48–72 hours after the scan. This is because of a potential harmful reaction from the medications and IV dye. Some physicians prefer that this exam be done after drinking a chalky oral dye to better differentiate your intestine from parts of your urinary tract. The pros of CT include the detailed images that it provides in addition to the relatively short amount of time it takes to perform the exam. Its cons are the risk of radiation exposure to the developing child in a pregnant woman and risk of an allergic reaction to IV dye.

Magnetic resonance imaging, or MRI, is one of the newest imaging modalities in use. The images that it provides are very detailed, and MRI has the added advantage of obtaining these images without the use of radiation. However, it does take a lot longer than the imaging modalities previously mentioned and is quite expensive. MRIs are performed when you lay on a small table and are passed through a small tube, which is actually a collection of very strong magnets. Because of this, it is very important to remove all metal objects and jewelry before this exam. If you have a fear of small spaces and become anxious at the thought of them, you may be given a small dose of an anti-anxiety medication before the exam. There are two types of MRI machines currently in use: open ones, which are more comfortable, and closed ones.

Although MRIs are wonderful tests that provide a great view of the urinary system, there are a few risks. If you have an aneurysm clip from a prior brain procedure, you must let your doctor know because this clip could become dislodged during the exam. No one with a cardiac pacemaker should have an MRI performed. If you have any type of implanted device such as an electrical stimulator or pump, you should not have an MRI performed. Pregnant women during the first trimester should not have an MRI; neither should metal or machine workers who may have a small fragment of metal in their eye. Contrast is sometimes given during MRI exams and patients rarely experience allergic reactions to it. MRI pros include detailed imaging and a lack of radiation. Its cons are its expense and patient discomfort due to claustrophobia.

Any of the previously mentioned exams may be ordered during your workup. As mentioned before, it is extremely important that you bring copies of the actual images with their accompanying reports to your first appointment with members of your bladder cancer team.

BLADDER CANCER GRADING AND STAGING

Cancer grade and stage are two terms you will most likely hear about during the course of treatment. Bladder cancer grade and stage are not the same and should not be used interchangeably to describe your cancer. Grade, expressed as a number, is used to describe the appearance of cells under the microscope and increases from 1 to 4 depending on how they look compared with normal cells. Grade of cancer refers to the aggressiveness of the disease. Grade 4 cancers are typically more aggressive than grade 1 cancers, and they recur more often. Cancer staging describes the extent or spread of the disease at the time of diagnosis. It is essential in determining the choice of therapy and in assessing prognosis. Cancer stage is based on the size and location of the primary tumor and whether it has spread to other areas of the body.

Table 1-2   Bladder Cancer Staging

Primary tumor (T)
TX: Primary tumor cannot be assessed
T0: No evidence of primary tumor
Ta: Noninvasive papillary carcinoma
Tis: Carcinoma in situ (i.e., flat tumor)
T1: Tumor invades subepithelial connective tissue

T2: Tumor invades muscle
    pT2a: Tumor invades superficial muscle (inner half)
    pT2b: Tumor invades deep muscle (outer half)

(continues)

Table 1-2   Bladder Cancer Staging Cont'd.

Primary tumor (T) *Continued*

T3: Tumor invades perivesical tissue
    pT3a: Microscopically
    pT3b: Macroscopically (extravesical mass)

T4: Tumor invades any of the following: prostate, uterus, vagina, pelvic wall, or abdominal wall
    T4a: Tumor invades the prostate, uterus, vagina
    T4b: Tumor invades the pelvic wall, abdominal wall

Regional lymph nodes (N)
NX: Regional lymph nodes cannot be assessed
N0: No regional lymph node metastasis
N1: Metastasis in a single lymph node 2 cm or smaller in largest dimension
N2: Metastasis in a single lymph node larger than 2 cm but 5 cm or smaller in largest dimension; or multiple lymph nodes 5 cm or smaller in largest dimension
N3: Metastasis in a lymph node larger than 5 cm in largest dimension

Distant metastasis (M)
MX: Distant metastasis cannot be assessed
M0: No distant metastasis
M1: Distant metastasis

The staging system used to describe bladder cancer in the United States was adopted by the American Joint Committee on Cancer in 2002. It is often referred to as the "TNM staging system" and it assesses tumors in three ways: extent of the primary tumor (T), absence or presence of regional lymph node involvement (N), and absence or presence of distant metastases (M). Please refer to **Table 1-2** for a description of the various bladder cancer stages.

If cancer cells are present only in the layer of cells where they developed and have not spread, the stage is called "in situ," meaning "in position," or not extending beyond the original site. If cancer cells have spread beyond the original layer of tissue, the cancer is invasive. Therefore bladder cancer is classified as either noninvasive or invasive, and each type is treated differently.

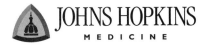

CHAPTER 2

MY TEAM— MEETING YOUR TREATMENT TEAM

WILMER B. ROBERTS, MD, PHD

PLAYERS: UROLOGIC ONCOLOGIST, MEDICAL ONCOLOGIST, RADIATION ONCOLOGIST, RADIOLOGIST, PATHOLOGIST, NURSES, AND OTHERS

With a new diagnosis of bladder cancer, many people in the medical community are on your side—your oncology team, all helping you to be well again. Each team member has a specific role related to bladder cancer and its treatment. The major players are as follows:

- *Urologic oncologist.* This doctor specializes in bladder cancer and performs surgery for it—cystoscopy, bladder biopsy, transurethral resection of a bladder tumor, examination under anesthesia, cystectomy, and partial cystectomy. We explain these procedures in detail in a moment. A urologic oncologist is a surgeon with expertise in the treatment of urological cancers. They will have completed a urology residency and will frequently have completed a fellowship in advanced cancer surgery (urologic oncology fellowship). This is usually the first doctor you see when referred because of suspicion for or a new diagnosis of bladder cancer.

- *Medical oncologist.* This is someone who specializes in bladder cancer and determines which medicines are appropriate for systemic treatment of the bladder cancer, if necessary. This systemic therapy may include chemotherapy after surgery (adjuvant chemotherapy) and/or chemotherapy given before a planned operation (neoadjuvant chemotherapy). The medical oncologist may consult with you before your surgery if certain clinical features suggest you would likely benefit from neoadjuvant chemotherapy, or the medical oncologist will see you (usually 1–2 weeks) after your surgery is completed when final pathology results are available if pathological features suggest a need for and potential benefit from adjuvant chemotherapy. A medical oncologist may also use chemotherapy to treat you if cancer recurs following surgery (salvage chemotherapy).

- *Radiation oncologist.* This person specializes in bladder cancer and provides recommendations about radiation therapy. This consultation usually takes place after your surgery and when pathology information is available. You may also see a radiation oncologist if you are not a candidate for radical cystectomy or if you do not want to have a radical cystectomy for your bladder cancer. In this case, radiation is frequently used in combination with chemotherapy to treat your disease.

- *Radiologist.* This is someone who specializes in imaging of the body using x-rays and scans (like CT or MRI scans). The radiologist performs these tests to adequately provide diagnostic information to accurately stage (or provide information that describes the extent of involvement) of one's body with cancer.

- *Pathologist.* Though you may never meet this person, the pathologist is one of the most important people on your team. The pathologist looks under the microscope at the tissue from your biopsy and from your bladder cancer surgery tissue to determine the extent of involvement of the tumor, whether cancer has spread to the lymph nodes, and provides important prognostic information that is used to determine your treatment plan.

- *Nurses.* Several nurses will assist your moment-to-moment needs as you journey through your treatment. Before, during, and after surgery; during chemotherapy; through radiation therapy; and even long-term care outside of the hospital, nurses provide education, assess your clinical needs, administer medications, and evaluate your progress.

- *Social worker.* This is someone who specializes in gathering the support services you may need and addresses financial concerns you may have about your treatment.

WHAT TESTS NEED TO BE RUN?

With a new diagnosis of bladder cancer, several tests need to be completed. Initially, your urine may be sent to a pathologist, who looks for the presence of cancer cells. Then, imaging of your body using a CT or MRI of the abdomen and pelvis and an x-ray or CT of your chest will be performed and read by the radiologist to discern whether the cancer has spread outside of the bladder. Next, a cystoscopy (a surgical procedure done under anesthesia to look at the cancer inside the bladder using a small-caliber telescopic camera) with biopsy, often with resection (removal), of the bladder cancer is performed. The material from the biopsy is sent to the pathologist for microscopic determination of the grade (aggressiveness of the cancer cells) and stage (extent of involvement of your bladder with tumor). While under anesthesia, a physical examination (called an EUA – examination under anesthesia) is done to assess the cancer in the bladder. This provides the surgeon with clues as to his or her ability to successfully remove the cancer at the time of definitive surgical treatment of your bladder cancer. Blood is also taken to assess your overall health and physiological preparedness for surgery. Additionally, consultations with the anesthesiologist, your primary care physician, a cardiologist, or other medical professional may be required. They will request any additional tests they believe are appropriate to ensure your preparedness for, and safety during, surgery.

YOUR INITIAL APPOINTMENT

The first person you will meet with a new diagnosis of bladder cancer is your urologic oncologist. When you call to make the appointment, you will be asked whether or not a surgeon (usually a urologist) has already performed a biopsy to confirm that you indeed have bladder cancer. If they have, you will be asked to bring with you (or have sent to the urologic oncologist's office) the glass slides of the actual pathological material taken at the time of the biopsy for review by another pathologist. You will also be asked for the written report of the original pathologist's interpretation of your biopsy material, all images taken in evaluation of your bladder cancer (either on CD or printed film) along with the written report of their interpretation, and any surgical operative notes from procedures performed by surgeons seen in the initial evaluation and diagnosis of your bladder cancer.

Be sure to obtain the address and clear directions, if necessary, of specifically where you are to go and what time you are to be at your initial appointment. If you haven't been to the facility before, allow yourself extra drive time to find it, find parking, and get to the location where the doctor will be. Being late only frustrates and distracts you from your ultimate goal of determining the treatment to help you arrive at your desired outcome. Bring the information requested above to ensure that your visit is as productive and efficient as possible for you and the doctor who will be seeing you. Often, the urologic oncologist or his or her office may have requested that the pathology slides be sent in advance with the goal that his or her urological pathologist can look at them before your arrival and render an opinion about the accuracy of the information provided in the typed report that you will bring from the outside evaluation. It is also helpful to know in advance if your insurance company requires you to get preauthorization for having additional tests done, such as a CT or MRI. There are situations in which the urologic oncologist, once he or she has reviewed the films, may find them inadequate. If this occurs, he or she may want to get additional imaging done while you are there for this visit. It is also likely the urologic oncologist will want you to leave your imaging studies with them to be reviewed by a radiologist. The imaging studies performed on your behalf are your property, but your urologic oncologist may need to retain them for use during your surgical care. Once the surgery and associated care for your bladder cancer is completed, the imaging studies can be returned.

It is helpful if you bring a trusted family member or friend with you. When stressed, we often only hear and retain some of the information that is discussed. You may feel overwhelmed, and the urologic oncologist will have a lot to explain to you. Trying to keep it all straight in your mind can be difficult. Bringing someone with you is helpful in that respect, and they may help you to feel a little more comfortable.

Also, bring an accurate list of ongoing and past medical problems, surgeries you have had, medications you are taking (including vitamins and herbs), allergies to medications or foods you may have, and your family history of cancers, heart disease, diabetes, lung disease, and other serious illnesses. This information may prove important for your medical summary and may influence some decision-making and treatment recommendations specific to you.

Having a list of questions prepared in advance is also helpful in making the time you spend with the doctor optimal and as efficient as possible. A list of some questions that may assist you in making the best and most informed decision for your treatment includes:

1. What type of therapy would you recommend for my stage and grade of bladder cancer?

2. What are common complications or difficulties that I should expect from the recommended therapy?

3. How soon would my surgery be scheduled?

4. What educational information do you offer to prepare me for surgery and what to expect?

5. Are there patients who had the same surgery done here and had a similar treatment plan that would be willing to speak to me?

6. Who will be my contact here for questions that arise?

7. Are there educational materials that you would recommend for other family members, like my children?

8. How many of the recommended types of bladder cancer surgeries do you perform a year?

9. What qualifications do you have to perform this type of surgery? Where did you do your residency? Did you do a fellowship in urologic oncology? Are you board certified?

10. Who else will be involved in my care and when will I meet them?

11. Do you anticipate I will need chemotherapy or radiation therapy and if so why?

12. Am I a candidate for, and would I benefit from, neo-adjuvant chemotherapy?

13. How often will I be seeing you after my surgery for ongoing evaluation?

14. Are there any clinical trials that you would recommend for me to consider at this point?

HOW BEST TO CONTACT TEAM MEMBERS

Request business cards from each healthcare provider you see and ask what their office procedure is for responding to questions/concerns you may have. Many of the phone numbers for the offices of the team members are available on the appropriate institutional or hospital Web sites. Usually, there is one contact person (a nurse or administrative assistant) who will make appointments and may be able to address some specific questions for you.

Once you have had an initial consultation with one of the bladder cancer team members, some of the team members may even prefer communication by e-mail. If this is convenient for you, it may be an efficient way to address critical (but nonemergent) issues that may arise between your appointments. Therefore if you have questions, please be succinct and think through the questions you may have as a courtesy to the team member for the time they must spend outside of an appointment in addressing your concerns.

NAVIGATING APPOINTMENTS

Calls initially made to a urology office or clinic are triaged by the scheduling staff who are trained to inquire about the current stage of your workup for your bladder cancer. It is most helpful to have a working knowledge of the tests and diagnoses you have already been given to best facilitate this process. The staff will schedule your initial appointment and mail you all necessary instructions before your appointment. After your initial appointment, subsequent appointments may often be arranged by the individual team members' staff over the phone. If at the initial appointment it is determined you should have a consultation with another team member (e.g., medical oncologist or radiation oncologist), that appointment is often arranged for you on the day of your initial consultation with the urologic oncologist—before you leave the clinic if you choose. Therefore having your schedule available allows you to efficiently make these arrangements without conflict.

FINANCIAL IMPLICATIONS OF
TREATMENT/INSURANCE CLEARANCE

You probably never planned on getting diagnosed with bladder cancer. There is no convenient time to get this disease, and the diagnosis alone can be difficult to manage. You will need to take time off from work and other duties for your surgery and possibly for other treatment afterward. It is helpful then to "get your ducks in a row" early on. Finding out how much sick leave you have, short-term disability coverage, copayment information, prescription coverage, and other medical expense issues is helpful to plan for the changes this will have on your budget. Your insurance company may require referrals to be obtained to see certain specialists, to get tests done, to get surgery authorized, as well as to obtain other treatments. If you need help with these things, ask for a social worker to assist you. Financial coordinators are available in the clinic. They will work with you to help you navigate the financial aspect of this process.

Some treatments may be recommended that involve participation in a clinical trial. Usually, a research nurse will assist you with navigating the financial aspects of this line of therapy and can provide much of that information for you.

If you lack health insurance, all is not lost. There are resources available for those who need help and meet certain criteria for financial assistance and coverage of their bladder cancer treatment expenses. Some states even have special grants for residents for precisely this purpose. Check with the social worker at the facility where you are being treated to get assistance and referrals. There are also organizations that provide support for transportation to and from treatment visits, provide food for you and your family, and even assist with coverage of some medications. They aren't available in every state so rely on the social worker to tell you more about what is available for your geographical area.

Financial support services are not well advertised. It requires you to take the initiative to ask about them rather than waiting for someone to tell you about them. Be assertive and do this for yourself. That's why these programs exist. Money is the primary reason family members get into arguments. Avoid this up front by discussing the issue and planning a budget. Be proactive in asking to meet with the social worker to discuss what support services are available for you as well.

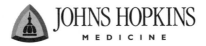

CHAPTER 3

JOHNS HOPKINS

M E D I C I N E

TAKING ACTION— COMPREHENSIVE TREATMENT CONSIDERATIONS

THOMAS J. GUZZO, MD

In this chapter we discuss the various treatments associated with bladder cancer. Bladder cancer treatment can include surgery, chemotherapy, radiation therapy, and immunotherapy. Although some of these treatments are used alone, often a combination of several treatments (i.e., both chemotherapy and surgery) is used for the most success. Selection of the most appropriate treatment is based on clinical staging, including pathological and radiographic information, and individual preference in close consultation with your physician. When choosing a bladder cancer treatment, it is important that you consider not only the potential for cancer cure but also the side effects and quality of life impact of various treatments.

SURGICAL TREATMENT

Surgery plays an important role in both the staging and subsequent treatment of bladder cancer. Transurethral resection of a bladder tumor (TURBT) is the initial treatment step in the vast majority of patients with bladder cancer. TURBT provides valuable staging information, and pathological results from these procedures are used to make further decisions regarding what, if any, additional therapy is needed. The gold standard treatment for muscle-invasive bladder cancer is radical cystectomy (removal of the bladder). Advances in surgical technique and anesthesia have reduced the complications associated with this procedure in the last two decades. The development of continent urinary diversion, which allows one to empty the bladder through the urethra, is an option for certain patients. Minimally invasive procedures such as laparoscopic or robotic-assisted radical cystectomy may also be treatment options. In addition, bladder-sparing procedures (either with partial removal of the bladder or aggressive TURBT frequently in combination with chemotherapy and/or radiation therapy) have allowed some patients to treat their cancer while leaving their bladders intact. Advances in surgical techniques continue to this day with the development of minimally invasive approaches to cystectomy. Both robotic-assisted and laparoscopic radical cystectomy have been performed safely in highly specialized centers and have the potential for decreased morbidity and a shorter period of recovery, but longer term follow-up is needed to determine if these procedures are equivalent to open surgical techniques.

TRANSURETHRAL RESECTION

TURBT is often the first procedure you will have once diagnosed with a bladder tumor. This surgery is typically performed under general or spinal anesthesia as an outpatient procedure and without any incision, endoscopically through the urethra, which means a cystoscope is placed through the urethra and into the bladder. Through this scope your urologist can see the inside of your bladder and has the ability to resect, or remove, tumors in the bladder under direct vision using electrocautery. The electrocautery is also used to control bleeding after the resection is completed. TURBT is extremely important for the staging of bladder tumors but can also be therapeutic for lower stage bladder cancers. Once the tumor has been removed, it can be analyzed under the microscope by a pathologist. The pathological findings dictate further treatment decisions. If the tumor is low grade and noninvasive, you will likely not need any further therapy at this point except for close follow-up.

By and large, you can expect to go home the same day that this procedure is performed. Depending on the extent and depth of resection, your urologist may decide to send you home with a Foley catheter in place for a few days to allow time for your bladder to heal. Generally, this procedure is well tolerated, but it is not uncommon to see blood in the urine for several days after the procedure. Many patients also experience lower urinary tract symptoms, including painful urination, frequency, and urgency for up to several weeks following the procedure.

RADICAL CYSTECTOMY WITH
PELVIC LYMPH NODE DISSECTION

Radical cystectomy is the gold standard treatment for muscle-invasive bladder cancer and is also the procedure of choice for individuals with high-grade recurrent bladder tumors. Radical cystectomy has proven to provide excellent long-term cancer-free survival in individuals whose bladder cancer has not spread beyond their bladders or into their lymph nodes. Radical cystectomy is the therapy by which all other treatments are compared and judged.

Technically speaking, radical cystectomy for men involves removal of the bladder and prostate and also includes removal of the pelvic lymph nodes. In women, the bladder and typically the uterus, ovaries, fallopian tubes, and portions of the vagina are removed, although more recently surgeons have been moving toward preservation of some of these structures to improve quality of life. Because the main function of the bladder is to store urine that is made by the kidneys, a mechanism for diversion of urine outside of the body or storage of urine in a newly created reservoir must be performed in the same setting. Various types of urinary diversion are discussed below.

Traditionally, the surgery is performed through a lower abdominal incision in the midline from just below the umbilicus (i.e., "belly button"). Hospitalization for this procedure is generally between 5 and 10 days, and up to 6 weeks are needed for complete recovery. In recent years minimally invasive surgical approaches that replicate the technique of open radical cystectomy have been developed. Both laparoscopic and robotic-assisted radical cystectomies are currently being performed at highly specialized centers. The principles of the surgery are the same, but the procedure is performed through smaller incisions using laparoscopic instruments. Using robotic assistance, your surgeon is able to perform complex operations with higher precision, under magnification. These approaches offer the potential advantage of a shorter recovery time, less blood loss, and less postoperative pain.

A pelvic lymph node dissection should be performed at the time of your surgery. This involves removal of the lymph node tissue in the most common areas of bladder cancer metastasis (spread of the cancer). The pelvic lymph node dissection has two important roles: to stage the cancer and to guide therapy. Individuals who are found to have cancer in the lymph nodes at the time of surgery generally require additional therapy such as chemotherapy. Studies have shown that up to 30 percent of patients with disease-positive lymph nodes who undergo a pelvic lymph node dissection will be free of disease at 5 years. Although there is debate among urologists as to exactly how extensive of a pelvic lymph node dissection should be performed, there is no debate that one should be performed. Although a pelvic lymph node dissection can add an additional 30–90 minutes to your procedure time, there is little additional morbidity associated when performed by an experienced surgeon.

Regardless of the approach, anyone who undergoes a radical cystectomy will require a form of urinary diversion because the bladder will no longer be there to store urine. This can have a significant psychological and functional impact on an individual's quality of life. Patients are often hesitant to undergo definitive surgery because of the anxiety associated with long-term urinary diversion. There are two main types of urinary diversion: continent and noncontinent. Both forms require surgically removing a segment of bowel (most commonly the small bowel) from your gastrointestinal (GI) tract and plugging the ureter from each kidney into this segment of bowel to provide drainage of urine. Noncontinent diversions (ileal conduit) are those in which the piece of bowel is brought up through the abdominal wall to a stoma and the urine drains continuously into a drainage bag. This is the most common type of urinary diversion performed in the United States. This procedure requires approximately 8 to 10 centimeters (3 to 4 inches) of small bowel, which is far less than that used for continent urinary diversions. Although the obvious disadvantage of this procedure is its lack of continence and need for a continuous drainage bag, it has less short- and long-term complications than that of the continent diversion. An external urinary drainage appliance is very well tolerated and patients adapt to them very quickly.

Alternatively, a continent urinary reservoir can be reconstructed using small or large bowel. Unlike noncontinent diversions, larger segments (up to 60 cm [2 feet]) of bowel are configured into a pouch that can store urine. There are two main types of continent diversions: orthotopic and continent-cutaneous. An orthotopic continent diversion is one in which the newly reconstructed pouch is reconnected back to your urethra and voiding occurs in much the same manner as before cystectomy. Continent-cutaneous diversions use a small channel made of bowel that is brought up through the skin on the abdominal wall. Unlike the noncontinent diversions, this type of diversion does not constantly drain urine but instead collects it in the pouch. Several times a day a catheter is passed through this channel in the skin to empty the urine from the reservoir. Although these diversions allow for urinary continence, which most replicates normal function, they are associated with increased complication rates and require much more effort to maintain compared to the ileal conduit. Additionally, multiple studies have not shown that quality of life is significantly improved with continent diversion compared to noncontinent diversion.

Sexual dysfunction after pelvic surgery can have a major impact on quality of life for both men and women. In recent years radical cystectomy with the aim of preserving sexual function has been explored in both men and women. Patients with evidence of cancer invading through the bladder wall either on preoperative imaging or at the time of surgery are not ideal candidates for this type of procedure. In men this entails sparing of the nerves involved with potency that run along and underneath the prostate. In doing so, sexual potency may be preserved in a significant percentage of men. More recently, some surgeons have explored the possibility of preserving a portion of the prostate or seminal vesicles, which are traditionally removed at the time of surgery. Preservation of these structures also decreases the risk of erectile dysfunction after surgery by not damaging the nerves that run in close proximity to them. Preservation of a portion of the prostate at the time of surgery also may improve continence in men undergoing an orthotopic bladder reconstruction. Although nerve sparing can be performed with little risk of decreased cancer control in appropriately selected patients, prostate- and seminal vesicle–sparing surgery are more controversial because there is potential for an increased risk of cancer recurrence and also the potential for leaving undiagnosed prostate cancer behind. In women, sexual function preserving radical cystectomy has also been explored. This involves preservation of the nerves important in both clitoral engorgement and sensation. Preserving organs traditionally removed at the time of surgery, including the uterus, fallopian tube, ovaries, and portion of vagina, may also allow for improved sexual function after surgery. It should be remembered that the first goal of surgery is cancer control, and organ- and nerve-sparing procedures may not be appropriate in all cases.

Radical cystectomy is one of the biggest and most complex procedures performed by urologists. In addition to its complexity from a technical standpoint, you will likely have many questions not only related to cancer control but also to quality of life after surgery. Cystectomy can affect your quality of life from both an emotional and physical standpoint. After surgery, you may face specific physical adjustments to the urinary diversion, possible changes in sexual function, and changes in bowel habits and function. Specific side effects and complications related to cystectomy and urinary diversion are discussed in Chapter 4. An essential aspect to enhanced quality of life after surgery is to be proactive in the decision-making process before surgery. Ask your surgeon many questions before surgery, because knowing what to expect after surgery will ease this transition. A cancer diagnosis is a difficult time for anyone, and thoughts and questions will race through your head faster than you can remember them. Write them down as you think of them, so you can have a complete discussion at the time of consultation with your physician.

As stated previously this is a big surgery, and your surgeon may have you see other specialists before your procedure to ensure you are in the best medical condition to undergo surgery. You may be admitted to the hospital the day before your scheduled surgery for any remaining tests and to prepare your bowel for surgery. In the last decade, however, medicine has become increasingly more out-patient based, and many surgeons have eliminated the preoperative admission and have you report to the hospital the morning of surgery. Your surgeon will most likely have you only consume clear liquid on the day before surgery to clear out your GI tract, which allows for a technically easier urinary diversion and may also decrease your risk of complications. Along this same line, most surgeons will have you do some form of bowel preparation the day or two leading up to surgery. This is also used to cleanse your GI tract before surgery.

Immediately after surgery you will generally stay in the hospital 5–10 days. Postoperative practice varies from surgeon to surgeon, but most leave a small drain in the abdomen to monitor for leakage of urine from the newly created diversion and intestinal contents from the reconnected bowel. If there is no evidence of an internal leak, the drain routinely is removed at the bedside (with minimal discomfort) before discharge from the hospital. Your surgeon may also leave a nasogastric tube in for the first day or so after surgery. This is a tube that goes from your nose to your stomach and keeps your stomach decompressed, which prevents abdominal bloating and vomiting.

Generally, starting on the day after surgery you will be out of bed and with assistance from the hospital staff will start walking. It is very important to begin walking as soon as possible because it will make you feel better, will help with early return of bowel function, and will decrease the chances of developing blood clots in your legs and pelvic veins. You will also be instructed on breathing exercises while in bed and sitting to help expand your lungs after surgery and to prevent pneumonia. One of the major obstacles before discharge is return of bowel function and resumption of a regular diet. Your GI tract can be slow to return to normal function, largely related to the bowel work required for the urinary diversion. This will take time, and it is important to not force your diet too soon after surgery because this will increase your chances of nausea and vomiting. In general, your body will tell you when you are ready to eat.

Use your time in the hospital to learn as much as you can about your urinary diversion. Most centers in which cystectomies are performed have an enterostomal therapist with expertise in taking care of patients with urinary diversions. If you have a new ileal conduit, they will go over the general maintenance of the abdominal stoma and urinary appliance bags. This will make you more comfortable and confident in dealing with your diversion at the time of discharge from the hospital. Upon discharge from the hospital, your surgeon will give you precise instructions regarding physical activity, exercise, and resumption of sexual intercourse. It is important to follow these instructions carefully to ensure a smooth postoperative recovery.

If you underwent a continent urinary diversion, you will likely be discharged from the hospital with a catheter in the newly created reservoir to temporarily drain the urine until the reservoir is completely healed. If you have a cutaneous catheterizable diversion, a catheter is left in the catheterizable channel and a separate catheter is often brought out through a separate incision in the abdominal wall. These are temporary and generally removed 2 to 3 weeks after surgery. If you have an orthotopic diversion, a Foley catheter is generally placed in the diversion through your urethra. It is extremely important that you are careful with these tubes at home because dislodgement requires replacement and occasionally can lead to damage of your newly constructed reservoir. Mucus is often secreted from the bowel used to create your new urinary reservoir, and the nurses in the hospital will teach you how to flush your tubes with sterile saline before discharge to avoid mucous obstruction, which can lead to inadequate drainage.

PARTIAL CYSTECTOMY

Occasionally, a portion of the bladder involved with tumor can be removed while sparing the remainder of the bladder. In selected patients this allows for preservation of normal bladder function and continence and decreased complications because no urinary diversion is required. Unfortunately, only a small percentage of individuals will be candidates for such an approach—generally, patients with smaller, solitary tumors on the dome of the bladder. Individuals with multifocal tumors, large tumor, or carcinoma in situ are not candidates for this procedure. Recovery time for a partial cystectomy is generally quicker than that of a radical cystectomy, and hospital times tend to be shorter. A Foley catheter is left in place for 7–10 days to allow the bladder time to heal.

CHEMOTHERAPY

INTRAVESICAL CHEMOTHERAPY AND IMMUNOTHERAPY

The basic function of the bladder is to store urine. By directly instilling medications into the bladder, physicians have capitalized on this property of the bladder. By placing these agents into the bladder, these agents come into direct contact with the cancer cells. Intravesical (within the bladder) therapy is often used for patients with non–muscle-invasive bladder cancer. It can be used immediately after TURBT, as a single dose, to prevent recurrence of noninvasive tumors and is also used in the form of weekly outpatient administrations (usually 6 weeks at a time) to prevent both the recurrence and progression of bladder cancer.

The two basic agents that are used as intravesical therapies are chemotherapy drugs and immunotherapy agents. The most commonly used therapy in the United States is bacillus Calmette-Guérin (BCG), which is a form of immunotherapy. BCG is actually a vaccine that was originally developed for protection from tuberculosis. In the 1970s and early 1980s, it was noted to have intravesical effectiveness for the treatment of non–muscle-invasive bladder cancer. Although the exact mechanism of BCG activity is unknown, it works through local stimulation of the immune system. A Foley catheter is placed in the bladder, and then BCG is administered through the catheter into the bladder for 1 to 2 hours. Traditionally, BCG has been given once a week for 6 weeks to patients with high-grade non–muscle-invasive bladder cancer or to those patients with carcinoma in situ. Some studies have shown that routine maintenance instillations in addition to the traditional 6-week course may be more effective in preventing disease recurrence. BCG has proven not only to prevent recurrence of bladder cancer, but also to prevent progression to muscle-invasive disease and therefore is the first-line intravesical agent used in the United States.

In Europe, chemotherapy drugs like mitomycin C, doxorubicin, epirubicin, and valrubicin are commonly used as first-line intravesical therapy. These agents are not considered first line in the United States because several studies have shown improved effectiveness with BCG compared to these drugs. Furthermore, unlike BCG, which decreases the risk of cancer progression to muscle invasion, these agents have never been definitively proven to have any effect on tumor progression. They are currently considered second-line agents for patients who cannot tolerate, have a contradiction to, or fail BCG therapy. The exception to this is the use of mitomycin C as a single instillation immediately after TURBT, which has been shown to decrease the risk of bladder tumor recurrence in up to 40 percent of cases.

Intravesical therapy is performed on an outpatient basis and is generally well tolerated. Common side effects during therapy include irritative voiding symptoms like painful urination, frequency, and urgency during treatment. Each intravesical agent has its own side effects, and it is important that you discuss this with your physician before treatment. Specific side effects of intravesical therapy are discussed further in Chapter 4.

SYSTEMIC CHEMOTHERAPY

Systemic chemotherapy is an important part of the treatment plan for many patients with muscle-invasive and locally advanced bladder cancer. The first-line chemotherapeutic agent used for the treatment of bladder cancer is Platinol (cisplatin). Cisplatin is used most commonly in combination with other chemotherapy drugs because it has been found that the combination of medications is more effective than any single agent alone. The two most common combinations are methotrexate, vinblastine, Adriamycin, and cisplatin (MVAC) or gemcitabine and cisplatin. MVAC is an older and more extensively studied regimen, but gemcitabine-cisplatin has shown equivalent effectiveness to MVAC with fewer side effects, making it the preferred choice of many medical oncologists today. One important prerequisite to cisplatin treatment is normal kidney function. If your kidney function is impaired, your medical oncologist will likely choose other second-line chemotherapy drugs that will be less toxic to your kidneys.

Chemotherapy for bladder cancer is administered either before surgery (neoadjuvant chemotherapy) or after surgery (adjuvant chemotherapy). No study has directly compared the effectiveness of one approach over the other, and each approach has its advantages and disadvantages. Neoadjuvant chemotherapy offers the advantage of reducing the tumor volume before surgery, which may decrease the chance of having a positive surgical margin at the time of surgery. Because it is administered early (before surgery), it has the benefit of treating the cancer at a potentially earlier stage when the burden of metastatic disease is small. Finally, because surgery requires a significant amount of healing time, patients may be more "fit" for the rigors of chemotherapy before surgery. Several well-designed, prospective, randomized trials have demonstrated an improved survival in bladder cancer patients who undergo neoadjuvant chemotherapy. Neoadjuvant chemotherapy does have two main disadvantages. First, because our current clinical staging systems are not 100 percent accurate, a significant percentage of patients who may not need chemotherapy will be treated and subjected to its side effects. Second, upfront administration of chemotherapy may delay cystectomy in patients who do not respond to chemotherapy.

Adjuvant chemotherapy is administered after radical cystectomy. Giving chemotherapy after surgery offers the advantages of administration only to those patients who absolutely need it, and there is no delay in surgery, which minimizes risk of disease progression. The main disadvantage of adjuvant chemotherapy is a potential delay in chemotherapy for patients who need it while they are recovering from major surgery. Adjuvant chemotherapy has been less well studied than neoadjuvant chemotherapy, but studies have demonstrated its effectiveness in patients with locally advanced and lymph node–positive bladder cancer.

Regardless of what chemotherapeutic regimen is decided on between you and your oncologist, it will likely be administered in a standardized 21- or 28-day cycle. Over the course of the cycle specific drugs will be administered on specific days. Cycles are often repeated two to four times depending on the stage of disease and its response to treatment. These medications are given intravenously, generally on an outpatient basis.

Bladder cancer chemotherapy can be rigorous and is not without side effects and complications, which is discussed in Chapter 4.

RADIATION THERAPY

Radiation therapy is most commonly used in combination with other treatment methods (chemotherapy and TURBT) in bladder-sparing protocols. There is little evidence to suggest that primary radiation therapy as a single agent is effective in treating non–muscle-invasive bladder cancer. Though radiation therapy is moderately effective as a primary treatment for muscle-invasive bladder cancer, 50 percent of patients treated in this manner will eventually develop metastatic disease. Additionally, many patients treated only with radiation will ultimately require a salvage cystectomy for local recurrence. External beam radiation as a sole treatment method is not currently considered adequate treatment in the United States.

TRIMODAL THERAPY WITH BLADDER PRESERVATION

In recent years the combination of aggressive TURBT, external beam radiation, and systemic chemotherapy has become an attractive option for individuals who desire to maintain an intact bladder or for patients who cannot tolerate surgery. The trimodal combination makes biological sense because TURBT maximally debulks the tumor before radiation and chemotherapy. Chemotherapy not only treats the remaining disease but also makes the cancer cells more sensitive to radiation, which enhances the therapeutic potential.

Bladder preservation requires an integrated and cooperative approach from the patient, urologist, radiation oncologist, and medical oncologist. To achieve optimal success, individuals who are unlikely to respond to this therapy should be excluded, including those with evidence of cancer extending through the bladder wall (stage T3). Individuals who do not respond during the initial chemoradiation period are encouraged to undergo cystectomy. This is an important component of this approach, because those who do not respond early to bladder preservation may still be salvaged with early conversion to cystectomy. In highly selected patients, trimodal therapy has shown similar overall survival rates compared with radical cystectomy.

CLINICAL TRIALS

There are currently many ongoing clinical trials in the field of bladder cancer that will hopefully improve not only the survival outcomes for patients with bladder cancer, but also the quality of life of those living with bladder cancer. Clinical trials are an extremely important aspect in the treatment of many medical illnesses. In fact, many treatments you undergo today, whether it is for bladder cancer or another medical condition, were likely at some point part of a clinical trial. Your physician may approach you regarding clinical trials that are ongoing at his or her institution or near you. Don't interpret this to mean your condition is not treatable with the currently approved therapies; your physician may just happen to know of a trial that may be helpful to you.

There are many types of clinical trials; some deal with new medical or surgical treatments for bladder cancer, some with new imaging modalities for diagnosis and staging of bladder cancer, and some with the possible prevention of bladder cancer. If you are approached about a clinical trial it is important to know exactly what you are getting into before you enroll. Although there is generally a lengthy consent process, the best way to be informed is to ask questions of both your physician and the person running the trial.

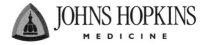

CHAPTER 4

BE PREPARED—THE SIDE
EFFECTS OF TREATMENT

THOMAS J. GUZZO, MD

It is important to remember that any treatment for bladder cancer, both surgical and nonsurgical, may be associated with complications and side effects. Some side effects can be mild and self-limiting, whereas others can more significantly impact your quality of life. The best way to plan for the side effects of treatment is to know about them ahead of time. Although this won't prevent side effects or complications, prior knowledge and preparation may ease any difficulties during or after treatment. It is also important to remember that each individual is unique and responds to treatment differently. If you know somebody who has been treated for bladder cancer in the past and had a particularly good (or not so good) experience, this does not necessarily apply to your situation. In this chapter we discuss some of the more common side effects and potential complications associated with the treatment of bladder cancer. The following discussion may seem overwhelming and a bit daunting, but its intent is not to cause you stress. For the most part, severe and significant complications with treatment are rare, but they do happen and you should consider your tolerance for such events when choosing the most appropriate treatment plan for you. The best preparation is knowledge; therefore being aware of potential side effects up front will allow you to make more informed treatment decisions.

SURGERY

Any surgery, regardless of how simple, has associated side effects and potential complications. As you learned in Chapter 3, a variety of surgical procedures are used for the treatment of bladder cancer, and all of them have their own unique side-effect profile. It must be remembered that surgery is not an exact science, and even a well-performed surgery by an experienced surgeon can have side effects and complications.

TRANSURETHRAL RESECTION OF A BLADDER TUMOR (TURBT)

Endoscopic procedures, including TURBT and bladder biopsy, are generally well tolerated and are performed on an outpatient basis. The most common complication after TURBT is bleeding. It is normal to see some blood in the urine for several days after the procedure, but a small percentage of patients have excessive bleeding after the procedure. It is often difficult for patients to differentiate significant bleeding from normal postoperative bleeding because a little bit of blood in the urine can look like a lot to the untrained eye. It is always best to err on the side of caution and discuss this with your physician if the amount of blood in your urine seems atypical to you or is getting worse instead of better. Passing a lot of blood clots in the urine is a sign of potentially excessive bleeding. If you do experience such a problem, don't panic. The vast majority of these cases are self-limiting and do not require any further surgical intervention. It is very rare to require a blood transfusion (unless you were anemic to start) even if you do experience bleeding after a TURBT. The biggest problem with bleeding after TURBT is the potential for urinary retention (inability to pass urine) due to obstruction from blood clots. Your urologist may admit you to the hospital and place a Foley catheter in your bladder to allow the clots to pass. Your urologist can irrigate the Foley catheter with saline to remove any residual clots. Rarely, if the bleeding does not resolve on its own, it may require a trip back to the operating room to cauterize any areas of bleeding from the prior resection site. This is done transurethrally, in the same fashion as a TURBT.

Roughly 5–10 percent of patients experience a fever after a transurethral procedure. This is almost always due to a urinary tract infection. The most common symptoms of a urinary tract infection in this setting are fever, chills, side pain, and frequent or painful urination. If you experience a fever postoperatively, you should contact your physician immediately. The vast majority of infections can be treated as an outpatient with oral antibiotics and resolve in several days. Most urologists give you antibiotics during your procedure and for a few days thereafter to prevent infection, but unfortunately a small percentage of patients will still experience an infection despite taking antibiotics. It is important to note that most patients have lower urinary tract symptoms after surgery. This is directly related to the manipulation from the cystoscope and any biopsies or resection that were performed. These procedures cause bladder and urethral inflammation, which may cause you to experience painful urination, urinary frequency, and urgency for several days after the procedure. These symptoms are very similar to that of a urinary tract infection and can be confusing, but they do not cause fever like a urinary tract infection. If you are unsure whether your symptoms are a result of an infection or the procedure, the safest bet is to consult your urologist as soon as possible.

Urinary retention (inability to pass the urine) is another uncommon and generally self-limiting complication one can experience after surgery. In men, this is often caused by swelling of the prostate due to manipulation from the cystoscope. Excessive bleeding may also result in clot formation that can obstruct the flow of urine. Patients who experience this side effect urinate in small volumes or not at all, even though their bladder is uncomfortably full. The treatment for this is simple; a catheter is placed in your bladder for a few days to allow any edema (swelling) to resolve. The catheter can then be removed several days later and most patients void without difficulty at that point.

At the time of TURBT, perforation of the bladder can occur. This happens if the full thickness of the bladder wall is resected at the time of TURBT. This is often inadvertent, but it can also be done intentionally by your surgeon in the case of a tumor that grows deep into the wall of the muscle. Most perforations are small and will close on their own, without additional intervention. You may need to have a Foley catheter for several days to permit healing and minimize leakage of urine from the perforation. In rare circumstances a bladder perforation may be so large or in such a location that it is dangerous to allow it to heal on its own. Such cases require open surgery to suture the bladder closed. This is performed through a lower midline incision. A Foley catheter again would be left in the bladder for several days to permit healing. Open surgery for bladder perforation is a rare event (less than 1 percent).

RADICAL CYSTECTOMY AND URINARY DIVERSION

Radical cystectomy and associated urinary diversion is a complex procedure. Even in the best of hands, the potential for side effects and complications is significant. The most common side effects and complications related to this procedure are discussed below. Although this will give you a good understanding of what to expect after surgery, it is very important that you discuss the risks of cystectomy with your urologist before surgery to be as fully informed and prepared as possible.

As with any major surgery, there is potential for bleeding during your surgery. Twenty-five to 50 percent of patients need a blood transfusion either during surgery or in the immediate postoperative period. Your surgeon may ask you to donate your own blood before surgery, so that it can be given back to you at the time of your operation. This is to minimize the risk of infection with transfusion-related bloodborne illnesses such as HIV and hepatitis. Because this risk is extremely low, many surgeons do not require you to donate your own blood. Your blood count will be monitored for the first several days after surgery because in rare circumstances bleeding can occur after surgery. Depending on your blood count at the time of discharge, your physician may send you home on iron supplementation.

There is a small risk of infection after surgery. Post-surgical infections can occur in the abdominal wound, intra-abdominally at the site of bladder removal, and also in the urine (urinary tract infection) or kidney (pyelonephritis). Most infections can be successfully treated with antibiotics. Wound infections can require a portion of your incision to be opened to allow drainage of infected material. This is easily done at the bedside and is not painful. Once the infection clears, the wound heals on its own without any further therapy.

Gastrointestinal (GI) complications and side effects are extremely common after cystectomy, mainly due to the bowel surgery that is required for urinary diversion. Anywhere from 30–60 percent of patients will have a postoperative ileus. Ileus occurs when there is temporary decreased motility of the intestine after surgery. Common causes of ileus are edema related to the bowel anastomosis, electrolyte imbalances and fluid shifts that can occur with surgery, anesthetic effects on the bowel, and retraction of the bowel at the time of surgery. The symptoms of ileus are abdominal bloating, decreased appetite, inability to pass gas, nausea, and vomiting with food intake. The treatment for ileus is to not eat or drink anything until GI motility returns. In doing so, abdominal distention, nausea, and vomiting can be minimized. Most cases of ileus resolve within a few days. Small bowel obstruction, which has similar symptoms to that of ileus, can occur early in the postoperative period or many years after your initial surgery. In this case there is an actual obstruction of the bowel, generally at the site of the anastomosis. Occasionally, this can be managed conservatively in much the same manner as described with an ileus, but often surgery is required to relieve the obstruction. Bowel habits can also change after cystectomy. This can range from constipation, to loose stools, to frank diarrhea. These symptoms are caused by the removal of the portion of intestine that is used for urinary diversion. As one can imagine, these symptoms tend to be worse in patients who have continent urinary diversions because larger segments of bowel are used. Many of these symptoms can be treated successfully with over-the-counter medications that either help with constipation or add bulk to the stool in cases of diarrhea.

There are medical risks associated with any major surgery, and cystectomy is no exception. These risks include deep vein thrombosis (blood clots in the legs), pulmonary embolism (blood clots migrating to the lungs), heart attack, stroke, and even death. Your overall health status going into surgery can increase your risk for certain medical complications. Your surgeon my require you to undergo a preoperative medical evaluation and clearance before surgery. This is very important because optimizing your medical status before surgery can minimize your risk for such complications.

Sexual function is often affected after cystectomy and is a major quality of life issue for both men and women undergoing this procedure. In men, the vas deferens (the tubes that carry sperm from the testicles) are cut, resulting in infertility. Although infertility is not a major issue for most men undergoing cystectomy, you should discuss this with your urologist before surgery if you are planning to have children in the future. Because the nerves responsible for erection are located along the base of the prostate, erectile dysfunction is a common side effect after surgery. In highly selected cases, these nerves can be spared at the time of surgery, leading to improved potency outcomes. Erectile function after surgery depends on three main factors: age, preoperative function, and nerve sparing at the time of surgery. Young men who have good erectile function before surgery are much more likely to have erectile function afterward than older men or those with preexisting erectile dysfunction. There are a variety of options to help with ED following surgery including the use of vacuum devices, oral medications (i.e., Viagra, Levitra, or Cialis), injection of medications directly into the penis, or a penile implant. In recent years there has been a trend toward preservation of the female sexual organs at the time of cystectomy, including the uterus, ovaries, fallopian tubes, and vagina. Such organ preservation strategies have also led to improved sexual function in women undergoing radical cystectomy.

There are both short-term and long-term complications associated with urinary diversion. In the immediate postoperative period, urine can leak from the site where the ureters were sewn into the bowel. This is generally self-limiting and heals on its own several days to a week after surgery. Very rarely is any intervention required. If you do have a urine leak after surgery, your physician will likely monitor this by the output of your drains that were placed at the time of the operation. When the drain output decreases, this is a sign that the leak has healed.

The majority of long-term complications patients experience after cystectomy are related to the urinary diversion. In fact, 10–20 percent of patients will need an additional procedure at some point over their lifetime to correct a problem with the urinary diversion. Over time, scar tissue can form at the site where the ureters were attached to the bowel, narrowing the lumen (cavity of the tube) that urine drains through. This is called a stricture. If a stricture occurs, it can inhibit the drainage of urine from the kidney, causing an obstruction. If this happens to you, you may feel pain in your back similar to that of a kidney stone, but some patients have no symptoms whatsoever if the stricture occurs slowly over time. Your physician will periodically evaluate your kidneys with CTs or ultrasound to ensure proper drainage. Treatment for anastomotic strictures involves opening up this narrowed area to its previous size to allow the normal flow of urine into the ileal conduit or urinary reservoir. This can often be accomplished endoscopically without intra-abdominal surgery, but if such conservative measures fail, open surgery with anastomotic revision may be warranted. Fortunately, anastomotic strictures only occur in 3–7 percent of patients, and open surgery for such strictures is even rarer. Similarly to the narrowing that can occur at the connection between the ureters and the bowel, patients with ileal conduits can experience narrowing of the stoma at the level of the skin, which can impede the drainage of urine into the bag. This is known as stomal stenosis. Although this can be managed in the short term by simply placing a catheter into the stoma to allow drainage of urine, a surgical procedure is often necessary to revise the stoma. This procedure can generally be done on an outpatient basis.

There are several long-term complications specifically related to the fact that urine comes in contact with the intestinal portion of the diversion. Metabolic complications, such as acidosis, can occur but are often not clinically significant. The risk for clinically significant acidosis is higher in patients with continent urinary diversion because there is more intestinal surface area that comes in contact with the urine. Your physician will periodically monitor you for metabolic changes simply by checking lab tests. The majority of metabolic disturbances can be treated with dietary supplementation. Five to 10 percent of patients with urinary diversion form urinary stones at some point in their life, and approximately the same number experience repeated bouts of urinary tract infection or pyelonephritis.

Continent urinary diversions have several complications that are unique compared with that of the ileal conduit. Patients with continent catheterizable diversion over time can experience leakage of urine from their catheterizable channel. Scar tissue can also form at the site of the catheterizable channel, causing difficulty with catheterization. Both problems generally require a secondary procedure to revise this portion of the diversion. Men and women with orthotopic urinary reconstructions can experience both urinary incontinence and urinary retention. The incidence of incontinence is greater in men than in women, but the incidence of urinary retention is greater in women. Urinary retention is often managed with clean intermittent catheterization, which consists of self-passage of a urinary catheter via the urethra several times a day to empty the diversion. If the idea of self-catheterization is unpalatable to you, this is something you should keep in mind when considering your choice of urinary diversion.

CHEMOTHERAPY

INTRAVESICAL THERAPY

Each intravesical (within the bladder) agent used for the treatment of bladder cancer has its own side-effect profile, but they all cause some degree of lower urinary tract symptoms during and for several weeks after treatment. These symptoms can vary from mild to severe from individual to individual and consist of painful urination, urinary frequency, and urinary urgency. These symptoms are very similar to a urinary tract infection but are actually caused by bladder inflammation and irritation from the intravesical therapy. Mitomycin C can cause a skin rash (usually on the hands) that generally resolves when therapy is discontinued. Although bacillus Calmette-Guérin (BCG) therapy is highly effective in treating non–muscle-invasive bladder cancer, some patients experience a certain degree of side effects related to treatment. Lower urinary tract symptoms can occur in as many as 80–90 percent of those treated. Less common side effects include blood in the urine, fevers, fatigue, and nausea. If you experience significant symptoms, your urologist can decrease the BCG dose, which makes treatment tolerable for many more patients. Because BCG is a live, attenuated vaccine (made from live organisms that have lost their virulence but still produce an immune response), it can cause severe infections in very rare circumstances. Infections associated with a high fever may require complete discontinuation of the BCG and antibiotic therapy for up to 6 months. When BCG is instilled into a patient's bladder who has severe cystitis, or after traumatic catheterization, it may be absorbed directly into the blood vessels causing a severe infection, called BCG sepsis. Fortunately, BCG sepsis is rare, occurring in less than 1 percent of those treated.

SYSTEMIC CHEMOTHERAPY

As discussed in Chapter 3, there are many different chemotherapy drugs and combination of drugs that are used to treat bladder cancer. Each drug has its own side-effect profile. A complete listing of all of these side effects is beyond the scope of this chapter. However, this section will summarize the general side effects that you may experience with chemotherapy. When discussing a particular chemotherapy regimen with your oncologist, it is important that you ask about the specific side effects of each medication so you know exactly what to expect over the course of your treatment.

Just as with surgery, the general side effects of chemotherapy can be broken down into short term (acute) and long term (chronic). The major short-term side effects of chemotherapy are nausea and vomiting, fatigue, loss of appetite, weight loss, hair loss, and reduction in various blood counts. The acute effects start shortly after administration of chemotherapy and can wax and wane over the course of your treatment. Often, over the course of your treatment you will start to feel better toward the end of a cycle as the side effects of the medication wear off. Dealing with the acute side effects can be physically and emotionally draining. You should discuss side effects with your physician and healthcare providers because they often have many tips to help alleviate such symptoms.

During the course of chemotherapy your blood counts will be closely monitored. Chemotherapy can cause decreases in many important blood cells, including red blood cells (anemia) and white blood cells (leukopenia). If your blood counts fall too low, you may require hospitalization. A significant concern with leukopenia is the increased risk of infection. Depending on how severe your leukopenia is, your physician may place you on antibiotics to limit infections and also give you certain medications to help promote the production of white blood cells. Similarly, if you become too anemic, a blood transfusion may be required to boost your red blood cell count. It is important to remain positive and remember most of these side effects resolve fairly quickly once your chemotherapy is completed.

Long-term side effects of chemotherapy include chronic anemia, neuropathy (nerve damage), sterility or infertility, and an increased risk of certain cancers. In most instances the chronic anemia resolves with time as your body recovers. If you are planning on having children, men should bank sperm before starting chemotherapy and women should consult their gynecologist about the potential risks of pregnancy after chemotherapy. Unfortunately, it is difficult to predict the course of neuropathy in many patients. Some nerve damage slowly resolves with time, whereas other nerve damage can be permanent. Neuropathic symptoms can run the spectrum from numbness and tingling, sharp pain, and burning sensations. There are medications to help alleviate these symptoms, and your oncologist may want you to seek consultation with a neurologist in the case of severe symptoms. Although it seems counterintuitive, chemotherapy may actually increase your risk for developing another malignancy. Fortunately, this rarely happens (likely only 1–2 percent of patients who receive chemotherapy). Your oncologist will be aware of such risks and will monitor you after treatment for potential recurrence of the primary cancer and for any development of secondary cancers.

RADIATION

Just like chemotherapy and surgery, radiation has both acute (during or shortly after treatment) and chronic (up to many years after treatment) side effects. Acute side effects from radiation include lower urinary tract symptoms, diarrhea, fatigue, bloody urine and stool, and decreased white blood cell counts. Decreased white blood cell counts tend not to be as severe as that seen with chemotherapy. The other symptoms listed above typically resolve with time after therapy, but some patients may experience intermittent bladder and rectal bleeding even years after their initial treatment.

Chronic side effects of radiation therapy include erectile dysfunction, occasional rectal bleeding or bloody urine, and decreased bladder function. In the same manner that

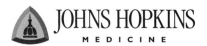

CHAPTER 5

STRAIGHT TALK—
COMMUNICATION WITH FAMILY, FRIENDS, COWORKERS, AND YOUR HEALTHCARE PROVIDERS

CHARLENE ROGERS, RN, MSN, AND

MARK P. SCHOENBERG, MD

A diagnosis of bladder cancer is overwhelming. You may ask yourself "Why me? What now?" In our practice we find that understanding the disease, your prognosis, the plan of therapy, and the details of what your care will mean are reassuring to you and your family. By learning about your problem, you can take control of it rather than it having control over you. For this reason it is critical to have a family member, a loved one, a companion, or a friend accompany you on the road to learning about this disease. Like any complicated problem, there is much to learn about bladder cancer, and having more than one head working on the problem makes the whole process easier for you. You will have to decide who from your circle of family and friends is best suited to make this journey with you. Having the support of a loved one through these troubled times is very important. You may not want to tell everyone about your disease until you are better able to come to grips with it. This will be a very emotional time for you, and you may feel you are on a roller coaster with your feelings. One day you will be fine, the next you may feel depressed. All of these feelings are normal, and keeping a positive attitude will help you endure the days ahead.

To come to terms with this disease, you will have to become a student again to some degree. We are surrounded by readily available information, but there are still enormous amounts of information out there to try to understand and comprehend. We often meet patients who have consulted the Internet and believe they are well prepared before their consultation. More often than not, these enthusiastic learners are frustrated by the complexity of information they have discovered and the difficult time they are having in making sense of their particular situation. Therefore before trying to do this research on your own, it is wise to first start with a frank discussion with your treating physician, the person who discovered your cancer: your urologist.

As a cancer patient, you may feel like a politician running for reelection. You may experience interest and concern (some welcome, some not) from many, and you will develop a personal strategy and style for dealing with three particular constituencies who are supporting your efforts in diverse ways: your advisors or professional healthcare providers; people who love you but may not depend on you, such as your friends and colleagues; and people who love and depend on you in some way, either practical or emotional, like your spouse or significant other, parents, and children. Let's talk about communication with healthcare professionals first.

Doctors, nurses, and other caregivers you encounter are just people too. Your relationship with the members of your team will mirror, in many ways, relationships you have in other parts of your life. Bring your natural courtesy and friendliness to the relationship and you are likely to get the same in return. Medicine is a service profession, and you should expect good service from your team members. However, unlike a restaurant or department store, a medical office may be forced to attend to the needs of customers who were behind you in line first if their problems require immediate attention. So, please bring your patience with you as well.

When speaking with your doctor and other team members, be as clear as you can be when it comes to how much you really want to know. Some patients want every detail, whereas others hardly want any information. Your cancer should not seem like an obligation to go to graduate school, but you should feel informed to your satisfaction. The amount of information is very personal, and you should make it known how much you really want to know.

Partner with your caregivers whenever you can. If something does not make sense to you, there is a reasonable chance that it does not make sense at all. Much of medicine is vocabulary, and learning the words that your team uses to communicate with each other will help you communicate with them as well. Does your doctor remember that you are allergic to penicillin? That you have a knee replacement? That you require antibiotics for a heart murmur before a procedure? Sure, but most professionals will be pleased if you help them remember these special details about you that affect your care.

Bring someone with you when you go for your consultations with your urologist. Two sets of ears hear more than one. Ask if you can bring a tape recorder and record the session so you can review it later at home. This also helps the concerned people in your life who could not accompany you understand the specific details of what your doctor is recommending. Make a list of questions to ask during the consultation. Print a copy for your doctor and present it to him or her at the beginning of the visit. This ensures that your questions are answered in a complete and unhurried fashion. Be sure that you ask questions as your care evolves. Ask if your doctor has other patients like yourself with whom you can discuss treatment and daily life. Talking to someone who has been where you are can be very helpful.

Talking to your boss, coworker, and friends is tricky and very personal. There is no rule on how to handle this part of your life. In most cases, you will want to let people at work know your diagnosis if it will significantly impact on your job. Most workplaces have clear-cut rules about this; in addition, make sure you are aware of the details regarding the Family Medical Leave Act so you and your family members can take advantage of this when appropriate. Hospitals have social workers to help you if assistance is needed. What you discuss with your healthcare team is private and protected by HIPPA (the Health Information Privacy and Portability Act). If you would like information shared with family or others in your circle, you must officially notify your doctor in writing. Most offices have a simple form you can fill out to facilitate this process.

Discussing your condition with your parents or your children is an emotional matter. These are people who love you and may actually depend on you, so they are interested in the success of your battle with bladder cancer. Cancer is a frightening concept, so the more calmly you can explain your situation, the more likely they will be able to provide you with support that is not compromised by the fear of the unknown. Teach them what you know, inform them of how they can obtain more information, and let them know you are getting the "best care." Adult children are in some ways the hardest to reassure. These grown-up kids, who may have kids of their own, look at you with a mixture of adult concern and childlike fear. You may want to ask your doctor to speak to them directly if you believe you are unable to satisfy their curiosity about your course of care. Your children may also push you to seek additional opinions, which is fine. We suggest you listen but don't let them push you around. This is your problem and you are the one who needs to feel comfortable with your healthcare team.

Talking with young children requires more finesse because they may not totally understand the disease and treatment options. You may just want to tell them you are sick and you are being cared for by your doctor. Reassure them that your doctor is taking very good care of you. Many children have heard the word "cancer" and become frightened. Please let them know that your illness is not their fault and they cannot catch the disease from you. Try to keep the routine at home the same if possible. Allow them to be included in your care on those "bad days." Perhaps they can bring you some water or something to eat. This small task will make them feel they are taking part in your care.

The Internet is a great place to get information as long as you know what you are looking for. In the past 5 years bladder cancer patients have seen two great sites dedicated to helping patients with this disease. The Web site sponsored by the Bladder Cancer Advocacy Network (BCAN, http://www.bcan.org) is a great source for basic clinical information

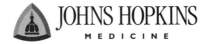

CHAPTER 6

MAINTAINING BALANCE— WORK AND LIFE DURING TREATMENT

KRISTEN A. BURNS, CRNP

There are various treatment options available for bladder cancer. A patient who has been diagnosed with noninvasive bladder cancer will have a different treatment plan from a patient diagnosed with muscle-invasive bladder cancer. Further details of each treatment and the impact of treatment on your life are discussed in this chapter.

Most bladder tumors are noninvasive. This means the cancer is localized to the upper layer of cells lining the bladder and has not invaded the underlying detrusor muscle. Once the cancer has spread to the bladder muscle layer, then it is considered muscle-invasive bladder cancer.

For patients with noninvasive bladder cancer, the tumor(s) is surgically removed during an operative procedure called a transurethral resection of bladder tumor. Because these tumors can recur, your doctor may prescribe intravesical bladder chemotherapy or immunotherapy to prevent a recurrence. Chemotherapeutic drugs, such as mitomycin C and thiotepa, work by destroying cancer. Because these drugs are administered in the bladder and not through the bloodstream, you will not have side effects typically associated with chemotherapy such as hair loss, nausea, vomiting, and fatigue. Immunotherapy, on the other hand, activates your own immune system to prevent the recurrence of bladder tumors. The exact mechanism of action is unclear. An example of immunotherapy is with bacillus Calmette-Guérin (BCG).

BCG THERAPY

HELPFUL HINTS

BCG requires 6 weekly visits to your urologist's office. Once you arrive at the office you will submit a urine specimen to make sure you do not have an infection or large amounts of blood in the urine. (If either of these is present, your treatment will be postponed until the following week.) A nurse will then insert a thin, flexible catheter into the bladder to empty your bladder of urine. After your bladder has been drained of urine a small amount (approximately 100 cc) of BCG is instilled into the bladder. You will be asked to hold the medicine in your bladder for 1–2 hours. Some urologists recommend you stay in the office for the duration of treatment, whereas others will permit you to go home after your BCG instillation. You may be asked to lie on your stomach for 15 minutes, lay on your back for 15 minutes, your left side for 15 minutes, and your right side for 15 minutes after BCG instillation. This allows your entire bladder to come in contact with the medicine.

After 1–2 hours you can empty your bladder, being careful to avoid splashing urine on the toilet seat or on your body and clothes, because you do not want to expose other members of your household to the vaccine. Men may find it easier to sit on the commode to urinate to avoid splashing urine. Wash your hands and genitals after urinating to prevent a rash or skin irritation from the BCG. To disinfect the toilet after you urinate, pour 2 cups of bleach in the commode and let it stand for 20 minutes before flushing. Follow this procedure for 6 hours after each BCG treatment.

Some patients may find it difficult to hold their urine for the recommended time after their BCG treatment. Scheduling your treatment for an early morning appointment and limiting your fluid intake before your appointment may make it easier to hold your urine. If you are on diuretics such as Lasix or HCTZ, take these pills after your BCG treatment. Most people will take the day off from work when they get their BCG treatment but will be able to return to work the following day.

Men can pass BCG to their partner during sex. It is important to wait 48 hours after BCG treatment before having sex and to wear a condom each time you have intercourse. Women should not become pregnant during BCG treatment and should also use a condom during intercourse. You should continue to use condoms for 6 weeks after your last BCG treatment. Once you have completed your 6 weeks of BCG therapy, your urologist will schedule a cystoscopy to examine the bladder for any residual tumor.

WHEN I MAY NOT EXPECT TO FEEL WELL

Common side effects of BCG include urinary urgency and frequency, burning with urination, blood in the urine, and flulike symptoms. Symptoms may start as early as 6 hours after your treatment and may last 1 or 2 days. Notify your urologist immediately if your symptoms last longer than 1 or 2 days or if you have fever, chills, joint pain, or cough. This could indicate the BCG has entered the bloodstream, causing a systemic infection and requiring the use of oral antituberculosis medicine.

CONTINUING WORK

You may continue to work during your BCG treatment. As previously mentioned, you may experience bladder irritability, frequency, and burning as early as 6 hours after your treatment, so you may consider scheduling your BCG appointment in the afternoon. This prevents you from taking a full day off of work for your BCG treatment and also prevents potential embarrassing frequent bathroom breaks at work. Scheduling your BCG treatment for a Friday afternoon is ideal.

INFECTION CONTROL

Any time a foreign object, such as a catheter, is inserted into the bladder there is a risk of urinary tract infection. Your nurse will administer BCG treatment under sterile technique to limit the risk of a urinary tract infection. Washing your hands after urinating and performing meticulous genital hygiene will also decrease your infection risk. Eating a healthy, balanced diet and taking a multivitamin will help keep your immune system strong.

SURGERY

If you have been diagnosed with muscle-invasive bladder cancer, the treatment of choice is radical cystectomy with urinary diversion. The ileal conduit is the most popular form of urinary diversion in patients with bladder cancer, but other options include continent catheterizable stoma (Indiana pouch) and orthotopic neobladder. Talk to your urologist to determine the pros and cons of each urinary diversion.

HELPFUL HINTS

Regardless of which type of urinary diversion you choose, being told your bladder must be removed is a difficult decision for most patients. Before choosing which urinary diversion is right for you, educate yourself by talking to your urologist, patients, family, and friends so you feel confident and positive about your decision. Being confident and positive in your preoperative decision helps to keep that mindset during your postoperative recovery.

You can expect to be in the hospital for 5–10 days (on average) following your surgery. The postoperative recovery can take 6 weeks or longer, so plan ahead of time and be sure to make appropriate arrangements for a leave of absence if you are employed. During this time period, you will be able to walk and perform light duties, but you should not do any heavy lifting or straining (no lifting more than 10 pounds). You will be working with a team of physicians, nurses, physical therapists, and enterostomal nurses during your recovery. The healthcare team will provide a safe environment and the necessary tools to support your recovery, but you must be an active participant in the recovery process. Pneumonia and deep venous thrombosis are potential, but preventable, complications. Your nurse will instruct you on breathing exercises such as incentive spirometry, cough and deep breathing, ankle exercises, and getting you out of bed as soon as possible to prevent postoperative complications. Though these tasks may initially be uncomfortable, they are imperative to help ward off pneumonia and deep venous thrombosis.

You may find it helpful to have family members or friends available to support you during your recovery. Family and friends can provide a diversion and remind you of your life outside the hospital. Bring pictures of your family, friends, and pets, books, radio, and your favorite robe or pillow with you to the hospital. The more comfortable and supportive you feel in the hospital, the more you will be an active participant in your recovery.

You will notice many tubes and drainage bags connected to you after your surgery. Your hand or arm may have 1 or 2 intravenous catheters (IVs) keeping you hydrated with intravenous fluid and providing pain relief with intravenous narcotics. Expect to have these IVs in place until you are tolerating food properly. There may also be a drain placed in your abdomen. This drain will be located in either your right or left lower abdomen and is typically removed before you are discharged from the hospital. Your surgical incision will be from your umbilicus (belly button) to your pubis. If you have an ileal conduit you will notice an ostomy bag on your abdomen to collect urine. These drains will be assessed daily by your physician and nurse.

You will be discharged home once you are eating a regular diet, passing gas and having bowel movements, and walking independently and your pain is controlled with oral pain medicine. A home health nurse may come to your house for two to three visits to make sure you continue to progress in your recovery.

CONTINUING WORK

Recovering from bladder cancer surgery is a lengthy process. It will take time to get your energy and stamina back to where it was before your cystectomy. You may initially find yourself taking more frequent rest breaks during the day. Listen to your body and rest when it is telling you to rest. Your energy will gradually return to normal.

You should avoid lifting anything over 10 pounds for 6 weeks to allow your abdomen sufficient time to heal. Because of this it is recommended you return to work no sooner than 6 weeks after your surgery. Because of the length of time you will be off work, you should inform your supervisor as early as possible with the date of your upcoming surgery and the convalescence time frame. Schedule a meeting with your human resources representative to verify you have the necessary forms completed such as Family Medical Leave Act or short-term disability.

INFECTION CONTROL

Your body and immune system may be weakened as you recover from surgery. Following good hand hygiene will help prevent postoperative infections. Make sure your nurse, nursing assistant, physician, visitors, or anyone who enters your hospital room washes their hands with either soap and water or an alcohol-based gel before entering your room. Hospitals carry many germs, and transmission can be prevented by simply following this simple rule.

Advise family members and friends to refrain from visiting you if they are ill or feel under the weather. A phone call will allow you to feel connected to your loved ones without worrying about possible infections.

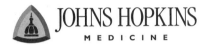

CHAPTER 7

JOHNS HOPKINS

MEDICINE

Surviving Bladder Cancer— Re-engaging in Mind and Body Health After Treatment

Joanne Walker, RN, MS, CWOCN

SURVIVORSHIP

What is a survivor? The dictionary defines it as one who remains alive or in existence or one who carries on despite hardship or trauma. The second definition certainly has more relevance here. Would we not all wish to do more than simply exist? A diagnosis of bladder cancer creates a degree of hardship because treatment in the form of chemotherapy, radiation, and/or surgery must be undertaken. This is not easy. Work schedules, family roles, and physical activities may need to be adjusted, at least temporarily. To carry on, the "survivor" must determine what treatment, adjustments, and sacrifices to undertake. Hopefully, the path chosen will be one that allows a full and rewarding life.

As a survivor you may feel isolated. To outsiders (meaning anyone other than the survivor) the stress appears to be over when treatment is over. You may compare it with going home with a new baby. The adrenaline that has been pumping and powering you through tests, chemotherapy, more tests, and surgery now drops and reality sets in. You think, "Now what do I do?" "Where is everyone? I need them now more than ever." "How will I be different? Will I be able to adjust?" There may be anxiety every time a routine follow-up test is due. You feel that nothing is routine; you wonder whether bad news is around the next corner. Part of you tries to focus on the positive: You are alive and able to live, love, and laugh, but the little bit of doubt that tickles at the back of your consciousness must be acknowledged.

It is helpful to start planning for survival as soon as a diagnosis is made. Think about how you have handled stressful situations in the past and recruit all the resources available to you, because this may be the greatest struggle of your life.

COUNSELING

It is not unusual, when faced with such life-altering circumstances, to find it difficult to maintain equilibrium. Doubt, anxiety, and depression may overwhelm you. You may recognize this yourself, or a friend or family member might speak to you of concerns that they have about you. Your doctor or nurse may recommend counseling. Short-term counseling may help you identify more effective coping strategies. Sometimes it is easier to discuss sensitive issues with a "stranger" rather than those who are close, as their emotional involvement may prevent them from seeing the situation objectively and identifying the kind of help that you really need. Just keep in mind that it is normal to have many conflicting or overwhelming feelings or to need help dealing with these feelings.

MANAGING LONG-TERM SIDE EFFECTS OF TREATMENT

Side effects of bladder cancer treatment are as varied as the multitude of treatments available. No matter what the treatment, time aids in adjustment and often improves the negative effects. For example, you may have encountered blood in your urine or stools after radiation or peripheral neuropathy, hair loss, difficulty concentrating, and/or fatigue from chemotherapy. If surgery was the option for you, adjusting to a bladder with reduced capacity or learning to care for and manage an external or internal reconstruction may present a challenge as you learn to incorporate it all into your normal routine.

It is difficult to be patient under these circumstances, but keep in mind you are learning new skills at a time when you are physically and emotionally taxed. It takes time. Set small, short-term goals for yourself.

LIVING A HEALTHIER LIFESTYLE

In many ways being a survivor of bladder cancer is a second chance at life—an opportunity to start new as a healthier, happier, more self-aware person.

NUTRITION

As we age it becomes even more important to be kind to our joints, backs, and hearts by maintaining a healthy weight. A low-fat diet rich in complex carbohydrates and protein is

79

favorable to healing and good health. Studies have shown that bladder cancer patients have lower levels of selenium and vitamins A, C, and E. We are learning more about the importance of vitamin D in the maintenance of bone health and decreased cancer risk. Chemotherapy sometimes causes a drop in vitamin D levels. Vitamin B-12 tends to decrease as we get older. The answer to all this is eating a diet as described above that incorporates fruits and vegetables. Vitamin supplements are helpful in maintaining therapeutic levels.

Adequate fluid intake (six to eight 8-oz glasses a day) helps you to stay well hydrated and may help to decrease your risk of urinary infection. All dietary supplements including cranberry should be discussed with your physician. This discussion should include all medications, including over-the-counter medicines and herbals that you are taking to avoid possible negative interactions.

SMOKING

As you know so well, there is a strong link between smoking and bladder cancer. In addition, smoking has negative effects on the heart, lungs, and circulation. If you are still smoking, consider joining a smoking cessation program or getting help with medication from your doctor. You will enjoy immediate benefits to your heart and lungs if you stop smoking.

EXERCISE

This helps maintain or achieve healthy weight, and the endorphins that are produced help to ward off depression. Return to your normal exercise routine as soon as you are allowed, or think about starting some sort of toning exercise program. Walking is a perfect start and can increase in speed and duration as you improve aerobically. You do not need to join a gym to exercise. Park a little farther from your destination, join a friend for "mall walking," or take the family dog for a romp.

STRESS

It is easy to say "avoid stress," but not so easy to do. Many aspects of your life that may have been put on hold for the duration of treatment now cry out for attention. Family and work responsibilities are waiting. This is, however, a good time to reestablish priories—to decide what is really important and what is not worth the worry. Eliminate what can be eliminated: Simplify your life and try to carve out some time for yourself. Take the vacation that you were putting off for "someday"; take a painting class, dance lessons—whatever you want! It is your life to *live*, and you have certainly earned a few rewards for yourself. Before your cancer diagnosis it was not so easy to say "no"—now, you can use that new perspective you have developed to stop and smell the roses.

SETTING NEW GOALS

Many times in life things happen that cause you to relook at the picture and change your course a bit. Maybe it is an important birthday, the death of a loved one, or the birth of a grandchild. There are few events, however, that are as life altering as a diagnosis of cancer. It may be the first time you consider your own mortality or think about the world without your presence in it. But, like George Bailey, with consideration you discover "It's a wonderful life." You realize that you have what few people do—a second chance. A chance to decide that it is never too late to have a positive impact in the world, to leave a legacy for your descendants and, if you are especially lucky, for those beyond your immediate circle of friends and family. You may decide that you do not want to spend your life working or that you *can* afford to try that "fun" job that you have always dreamed about.

Your family and friends may have some difficulty understanding the changes in you. Communication is key. You may wish to seek advice from those who have "been there." Find a support group in your area. Many hospitals have them. Some hospitals have support groups specifically for cystectomy patients, and the oncology resources of a Cancer Center can provide many avenues for support and expression for those with a cancer diagnosis.

SEEING THE WORLD THROUGH DIFFERENT EYES

As we discussed above, you may set new goals as you discover that you have a new perspective on life. You have rediscovered the "splendor in the grass, the glory in the flower"—it is natural to want to share your joy. One way is to be a mentor for other bladder cancer patients. As you remember how lonely and frightened you felt in the beginning, you may choose to ease that path for your fellows. Simply talking to someone who has "been through it" can do much to alleviate anxiety. Depending on how far out you are from your diagnosis, you may still benefit from a mentor yourself, someone who can help calm your fears or laugh with you about the bumps in the road. Your physical recovery may be completed months or years before your psychological and emotional recovery. You must acknowledge this and give yourself permission to feel however you *do* feel and you can decide what, if any, changes must be made.

A wonderful way to find positives in this experience is to involve yourself in education about this disease, whether in writing to your congressperson to ask for more research funding or speaking at a middle school about the dangers of smoking. There are many ways to make an impact. Remember, you *are* a survivor.

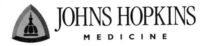

CHAPTER 8

MANAGING RISK—
WHAT IF MY CANCER
COMES BACK?

PHILLIP PIERORAZIO, MD

The bladder contains a number of layers, with muscle making up the deep layers and the bladder lining constituting the top layers. Up to 70 percent of bladder tumors are non–muscle-invasive at the time of initial presentation and may not represent life threatening disease. However, approximately 50–90 percent of noninvasive cancers will recur within 5 years of diagnosis and initial treatment. The likelihood of recurrence increases for patients who have high-grade tumors, large tumors, multiple tumors, flat tumors (versus tumors that grow on a stalk), or tumors that appear to invade small vessels that transport blood or lymphatic fluid. For that reason patients who have bladder cancer are monitored very closely and on a regular basis.

For many patients, knowing that bladder cancer is likely to recur can be associated with great anxiety. However, most of these recurrences can be managed with further transurethral surgery (resection of the tumors via cystoscope) or intravesical chemotherapy (medication placed inside the bladder) such as mitomycin C or bacillus Calmette-Guérin (BCG) therapy. For patients with low-grade (less aggressive) disease, 5–10 percent will progress to worse (or invasive) disease when they recur. For patients with high-grade bladder cancer (the more aggressive type), 15–50 percent will progress to invasive disease and 10–25 percent will die of bladder cancer. For this reason it is of the utmost importance for patients with high-grade bladder cancer to be monitored very closely.

PREVENTION AND MONITORING FOR RECURRENCE

The main tests used to monitor for bladder cancer recurrence are urine cytology and cystoscopy. The cytology test involves asking the patient to urinate into a cup, which is then sent to the laboratory where a pathologist examines it under the microscope. The presence of cancerous cells indicates that a patient most likely has bladder cancer. The absence of cancerous or suspicious cells does not necessarily rule out bladder cancer. Cystoscopy involves looking into the bladder with a camera and is performed by a urologist. Flexible cystoscopy refers to office-based cystoscopy, which occurs with a smaller, bendable camera without the need for general anesthesia. With flexible cystoscopy bladder tumors can be visualized; however, if there is a need to treat the tumors, cystoscopy often needs to be performed in the operating room.

Most urologists check urine cytology and perform flexible cystoscopy 3 months after the treatment for an initial diagnosis of bladder cancer. The timing of the initial check and subsequent follow-up depends on a number of factors. Intervals are usually 3–6 months and vary depending on whether the patient has low- or high-grade bladder cancer, if they received intravesical treatment, and the level of concern about recurrence based on the patient's risk factors and appearance of the first tumor. In general, patients with low-grade tumors are watched every 3–6 months for several years after initial diagnosis. Patients with high-grade tumors are followed with cytology and cystoscopy every 3 months for 2 years, then every 6 months for 2 years, and then annually thereafter is typically recommended. It is also suggested that the upper urinary tract (kidneys and ureters) are imaged (by x-ray, CT, or MRI) every 1–2 years to ensure that the tumors do not recur elsewhere in the urinary tract (outside of the bladder).

TREATMENT OPTIONS

Patients who recur with a positive cytology (cancerous cells present on urinalysis) and/or a suspicious finding on cystoscopy have many treatment options. These vary depending on specific patient characteristics and the overall situation. In general, if a lesion is seen during cystoscopy, it should be resected. If cytology is positive but no lesions are seen during cystoscopy or radiographic imaging, a patient can continue with close observation at 3-month intervals, undergo random bladder biopsies with cytology taken directly from the ureters, or start BCG treatment. After an initial 6-week course of BCG treatment, patients may sometimes continue with maintenance BCG treatment, which is believed to decrease the likelihood of bladder cancer recurrence; patients will continue to receive three weekly treatments of BCG on a regular basis (usually at

3 and 6 months, followed by 6-month intervals for a total of 3 years).

If chemotherapy was used first, BCG should be used as the second agent. If BCG was used initially, a second course of BCG can be repeated or BCG + interferon can be used as intravesical therapy. However, approximately 80 percent of patients who receive two courses of intravesical treatment will not have their bladder cancer controlled by medication alone. Therefore if a patient continues to recur despite continued resections and intravesical treatments, especially if they have high-grade disease, the risk of invasive disease continues to rise and they should consider cystectomy, which is surgical removal of the bladder. If they are unable or do not wish to undergo surgery, there are alternative therapies, including chemotherapy or radiation therapy. These therapies do not often control cancer as well as surgical removal of the bladder. If a patient recurs and the cancer has spread outside of the bladder, either by invading other organs in the pelvis or spreading to lymph nodes, there remain effective treatments to control the cancer. Options include surgery (cystectomy) in combination with chemotherapy and/or radiation.

If you have undergone radical cystectomy for treatment of your bladder cancer, your surgeon will continue to monitor for signs of disease recurrence usually with a CT scan at various time intervals (i.e., every 3 to 6 months). A CT scan is the primary imaging modality that is used to detect recurrent disease after surgery. If your cancer comes back following radical cystectomy, chemotherapy is frequently used for treatment. The use of anticancer medications to treat disease recurrence following radical cystectomy is called salvage chemotherapy. In certain cases, radiation and/or surgery may also be used to treat specific sites of disease recurrence.

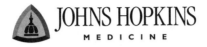

CHAPTER 9

JOHNS HOPKINS
M E D I C I N E

My Cancer Isn't Curable— What Now?

Charles G. Drake, MD, PhD

UNDERSTANDING METASTATIC BLADDER CANCER

Metastatic bladder cancer means that your cancer has moved beyond the bladder to other parts of your body. Hearing this news may be shocking, especially if you've gone through other treatments like surgery or radiation therapy with the idea of trying to cure your cancer. This is an important time to talk with your doctor as well as with your loved ones about what comes next. Although it might seem early, it's also a good time to make sure that your finances are in order and that your loved ones are aware of your wishes. It might also be a good time to think about whether you want to have an advanced directive, a legal document that tells how you want your medical care to proceed in the future. In general, metastatic bladder cancer is not a curable disease. Some patients live a long time on and off therapy, but, unfortunately, those patients are not very common. At this time the goals of your treatment will most likely change from trying to cure your bladder cancer to keeping it in check and to help you to live as long and as well as possible.

SHORT-TERM GOALS

Usually, the first treatment goal for patients with metastatic bladder cancer is to slow down the growth of the cancer. This is usually accomplished with chemotherapy, and your doctor will help you decide which type of chemotherapy seems most likely to help your bladder cancer. Chemotherapy can be difficult to take, and it's important for you to have a good relationship with your doctor and the nurses that administer your treatments. Most of the side effects of chemotherapy can be managed, but only if you share your symptoms and feelings with your treatment team. There are many kinds of medicines for each of the side effects that chemotherapy can cause, and often you can feel better just by switching to a medicine that works better for you. Patients with bladder cancer sometimes suffer from pain, and this is another symptom that you and your medical team should work hard to control. At this time it's natural for some patients to keep quiet about their pain and other symptoms because they believe their doctors will feel their cancer is getting worse. Keeping quiet is a bad idea, because it makes it much harder for you and your doctor to achieve a big part of your treatment goal—feeling as well as possible as long as possible.

Once you receive several chemotherapy treatments, your doctor will perform imaging and blood tests to see if the treatment is working. If the treatment is working and you are not suffering too much from the treatment, you and your doctor will usually plan on giving an additional set of treatments. On the other hand, the first treatment doesn't work in everyone, and if it seems to not have worked on your bladder cancer, you and your doctor will probably want to talk about trying a different kind of treatment if you are feeling up to it.

LONG-TERM GOALS

For patients with metastatic bladder cancer, it's very important to be realistic about the future. Because very few patients with this disease are alive 3 years out, it would not be smart for you to postpone planned vacations far into the future. If important family events like weddings or parties can be moved to an earlier time, it's a good idea to do so. But, it's also important to keep a positive outlook as well. Some bladder cancer patients with metastatic disease do very well, and you should be hopeful that you can be one of those. For some patients with bladder cancer, the disease becomes more like a chronic condition, and they go off and on chemotherapy as the disease grows and shrinks. This can go on for several years, but it's always important to keep in mind the idea of balancing the quality of your life with the amount of life you have to enjoy.

WHEN TO SAY WHEN

For some patients with bladder cancer, the treatments don't seem to work. For other patients, the treatments may work for a while but eventually fail. Although your doctor usually can find another treatment to try, there might come a time when you should think about stopping treatment. This is often a very difficult decision to make for both you and your doctor. If you believe it might be time to stop treatment, it's a good idea to have an honest discussion with your doctor.

Sometimes your family and loved ones will be helpful in coming to this kind of a decision, but sometimes it's better to have this discussion alone with your doctor. You should try to keep in mind that these kinds of talks are often difficult for doctors as well—doctors are trained to treat and to try and heal. But if the treatments are hurting you more than they are helping you, then it might be time to stop. Remembering the treatment goals of living as long as possible but as well as possible can be helpful in coming to a decision about when to stop cancer treatment.

PALLIATIVE CARE

When you and your doctor decide to stop treating your bladder cancer, this does not mean that you will stop trying to treat your symptoms. The goal of therapy at this time will shift to trying to help you to live as well as possible. Your doctor might call in a palliative care team, a team of experts who specializes in managing the kinds of symptoms that occur later in cancer treatment. This kind of team can be very helpful, because the members are often very experienced in helping you manage pain, tiredness, and other symptoms. Sometimes, it becomes difficult for a patient and their family to provide the best care, and your doctor might talk to you about entering a program called hospice. Hospice can be an in-home program, or you might move to a specialized care center. Like other palliative care, hospice care will help you to get the most out of the time you have left with your family and loved ones. Counseling may be provided to you and your family members, and your spiritual needs will be addressed. This is a time for you to reflect, spend time with loved ones, and gain a sense of peace.

CHAPTER 10

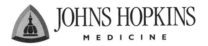

BLADDER CANCER
IN OLDER ADULTS

GARY R. SHAPIRO, MD

The risk of developing bladder cancer increases with age. The average age at diagnosis is around 70, but it is 10 times more frequent in those over 80 than in those younger than 80. As we live longer, the number of people with cancers of the bladder increases. In the next 25 years, the number of people who are 65 years of age and older will double, and the largest increases in cancer incidence will occur in those older than 80 years of age.

Older adults with cancer often have other chronic health problems and may be taking multiple medications that can affect their cancer treatment plan. Prejudice, misunderstanding, and limited access to clinical trials often prevent older patients from getting the timely cancer treatment that they need.

Older men and woman may not have adequate screening for bladder cancer, and when a cancer is found, it is too often ignored or undertreated. As a result, older individuals often have more advanced stage cancer and worse outcomes than younger patients. Older patients have less surgery and less adjuvant chemotherapy, and their metastatic bladder cancer is often left untreated.

WHY IS THERE MORE CANCER IN OLDER PEOPLE?

The organs in our body are made up of cells. Cells divide and multiply as the body needs them. Cancer develops when cells in a part of the body grow out of control. The body has a number of ways to repair damaged control mechanisms, but as we get older these do not work as well. Although our healthier lifestyles have allowed us to avoid death from infection, heart attack, and stroke, we may now live long enough for a cancer to develop. People who live longer have increased exposure to cancer-causing agents (carcinogens) in the environment (such as chemicals and tobacco, see Chapter 1). Aging decreases the body's ability to protect us from these carcinogens and to repair cells that are damaged by these and other processes. Inflammation also contributes to bladder cancer (see Chapter 1). Recurrent bladder infections and, in men, prostate problems lead to increased inflammation and may partially explain why bladder cancer is so common in older people.

BLADDER CANCER IS DIFFERENT IN OLDER PEOPLE

Compared with younger patients, older people with bladder cancer are likely to have a more advanced stage of invasive cancer. Tumor grade is also higher in older than in younger individuals, even if the cancer is superficial. Indeed, advanced age itself may be one of the main contributing factors in bladder cancer development.

DECISION MAKING: 7 PRACTICAL STEPS

1. GET A DIAGNOSIS

No matter how "typical" the signs and symptoms, first impressions are sometimes wrong. That blood in your urine or the difficulty that you are having urinating may well be due to a urinary tract infection or some other benign problem. Although most bladder cancers are urothelial (transitional cell), other types (primary or secondary) do occur, and their treatment and prognosis is often quite different. A diagnosis helps you and your family understand what to expect and how to prepare for the future, even if you cannot get curative treatment. Knowing the diagnosis also helps your doctor treat your symptoms better. Many people find "not knowing" very hard and are relieved when they finally have an explanation for their symptoms. Sometimes a frail patient is obviously dying, and diagnostic studies can be an additional burden. In such cases it may be quite reasonable to focus on symptom relief (palliation) without knowing the details of the diagnosis.

2. KNOW THE CANCER'S STAGE

The cancer's stage defines your prognosis and treatment options. No one can make informed decisions without it. Just as there may be times when the burdens of diagnostic studies may be too great, it may also be appropriate to do without full staging in a very frail, dying patient.

As it is in younger patients, stage is determined by the depth of the tumor, the presence or absence of cancer in lymph nodes, or its spread (metastasis) to other organs.

When doctors combine this information with information regarding your cancer's grade, they can predict what impact, if any, your bladder cancer is likely to have on your life expectancy and quality of life.

3. KNOW YOUR LIFE EXPECTANCY

Anticancer treatment should be considered if you are likely to live long enough to experience symptoms or premature death from bladder cancer. If your life expectancy is so short that the cancer will not significantly affect it, there may be no reason to treat your cancer.

However, chronological age (how old you are) should not be the only thing that decides how your cancer should, or should not, be treated. Despite advanced age, people who are relatively well often have a life expectancy that is longer than their life expectancy with bladder cancer. The average 70-year-old woman is likely to live another 16 years and the average 70-year-old man another 12 years. A similar 85-year-old can expect to live an additional 5 to 6 years and remain independent for most of that time. Even an unhealthy 75-year-old man or woman probably will live 5 to 6 more years, long enough to suffer symptoms and early death from recurrent bladder cancer.

4. UNDERSTAND THE GOALS

Goals of Treatment

It is important to be clear whether the goal of treatment is cure or palliation (radiation or chemotherapy for incurable advanced or metastatic bladder cancer). If the goal is palliation, you need to understand if the treatment plan will extend your life, control your symptoms, or both. How likely is it to achieve these goals, and how long will you enjoy its benefits?

When the goal of treatment is palliation, chemotherapy should never be administered without defined endpoints and timelines. It should be clear to everyone what "counts" as success, how it will be determined (for example, a symptom controlled or a smaller mass on CT), and when. You and your family should understand what your options are at each step, and how likely each is to meet your goals. If this is not clear, ask your doctor to explain it in words that you understand.

Goals of the Patient

In addition to the traditional goals of tumor response, increased survival, and symptom control, older cancer patients often have goals related to quality of life. These may include physical and intellectual independence, spending quality time with family, taking trips, staying out of the hospital, or even economic stability. At times, palliative care or hospice may meet these goals better than active anticancer treatment. In addition to the medical team, older patients often turn to family, friends, and clergy to help guide them.

5. DETERMINE IF YOU ARE FIT OR FRAIL

Deciding how to treat cancer in someone who is older requires a thorough understanding of his or her general health and social situation. Decisions about cancer treatment should never focus on age alone.

Age Is Not a Number

Your actual age (chronological age) has limited influence on how cancer will respond to therapy or its prognosis. Biological and other changes associated with aging are more reliable in estimating an individual's vigor, life expectancy, or the risk of treatment complications. These changes include malnutrition, loss of muscle mass and strength, depression, dementia, falls, social isolation, and the ability to accomplish daily activities such as dressing, bathing, eating, shopping, housekeeping, and managing one's finances or medication.

Chronic Illnesses

Older cancer patients are likely to have chronic illnesses (comorbidity) that affect their life expectancy; the more you have, the greater the effect. This effect has very little impact on the behavior of the cancer itself, but studies do show that comorbidity has a major impact on treatment outcome and its side effects.

6. BALANCE BENEFITS AND HARMS

Fit older bladder cancer patients respond to treatment similarly to their younger counterparts. However, a word of caution is in order. Until recently, few studies included older individuals, and it may not be appropriate to apply these findings to the diverse group of older cancer patients.

The side effects of cancer treatment are never less severe in the elderly. In addition to the standard side effects, there are significant age-related toxicities to consider. Though most of these are more a function of frailty than chronological age, even the fittest senior cannot avoid the physical effects of aging. In addition to the changes in fat and muscle that you see in the mirror, there are age-related changes in your kidney, liver, and digestive (gastrointestinal) function. These changes affect how your body absorbs and metabolizes anticancer drugs and other medicines. The average senior takes many different medicines (to control, for example, high blood pressure, high cholesterol, osteoporosis, diabetes, arthritis, etc.). This "polypharmacy" can cause undesirable side effects as the many drugs interact with each other and the anticancer medications.

7. GET INVOLVED

Healthcare providers and family members often underestimate the physical and mental abilities of older people and their willingness to face chronic and life-threatening conditions. Studies clearly show that older patients want detailed and easily understood information about potential treatments and alternatives. Patients and families may consider cancer untreatable in the aged and not understand the possibilities offered by treatment.

Although patients with dementia pose a unique challenge, they are frequently capable of participating in goal setting and simple discussions about treatment side effects and logistics. Caring family members and friends are often able to share the patient's life story so that healthcare workers can work with them to make decisions consistent with the patient's values and desires. This, of course, is no substitute for a well thought out and properly executed living will or healthcare proxy.

Although it is hard to face the possibility of life-threatening events at any age, it is always better to be prepared and to "put your affairs in order." In addition to estate planning and wills, it is critical that you outline your wishes regarding medical care at the end of life and make legal provisions for someone to make those decisions if you are unable to make them for yourself.

TREATING BLADDER CANCER

YOU NEED A TEAM

Cancer care changes rapidly, and it is hard for the generalist to keep up to date, so referral to a specialist is essential. The needs of an older cancer patient often extend beyond the doctor's office and the traditional services provided by visiting nurses. These needs may include transportation, nutrition, emotional, financial, physical, or spiritual support. When an older woman or man with bladder cancer is the primary caregiver for a frail or ill spouse, grandchildren, or other family members, special attention is necessary to provide for their needs as well. Older cancer patients cared for in geriatric oncology programs benefit from multidisciplinary teams of oncologists, geriatricians, psychiatrists, pharmacists, physiatrists, social workers, nurses, clergy, and dieticians, all working together as a team to identify and manage the stressors that can limit effective cancer treatment.

SURGERY

Though radical cystectomy is often complex, it is the gold standard treatment for high-risk patients whose bladder cancer has not spread to distant organs (see Chapter 3). Like other treatment options, surgery in some older individuals may involve risks related to decreases in body organ function (especially heart and lung), and it is essential that the surgeon and anesthetist work closely with your primary care physician (or a consultant) to fully assess and treat these problems before, during, and after the operation.

Surgery can be as effective in elderly patients as in younger patients, but it does have a higher rate of postoperative complications in older individuals who have other medical problems (comorbidities). Elderly people are particularly sensitive to long-term complications, like the metabolic disturbances that can follow urinary diversion (see Chapter 4).

In those aged 80 or older, the role of radical cystectomy is controversial. Although newer surgical techniques and improvements in care, before and after the operation, make this an option for increasing numbers of older patients, several studies suggest that its benefit is at best quite minimal, even in relatively fit octogenarians. You need to carefully weigh the benefits and risks of radical cystectomy with your multidisciplinary team before going through such an aggressive operation.

Early stage, noninvasive bladder cancers are treated (see Chapter 3) by the relatively low-risk transurethral resection of a bladder tumor that is usually well tolerated in all but the most frail individuals. Intravesical therapy also has few side effects in the elderly, but some studies suggest that the response to bacillus Calmette-Guérin (BCG) therapy may be decreased in those aged 80 years or over.

CHEMOTHERAPY

Nonfrail older cancer patients respond to chemotherapy similarly to their younger counterparts. Though the side effects of cancer treatment are never less burdensome in the elderly, they can be managed by oncologists, especially geriatric oncologists, who work in teams with others who specialize in the care of the elderly. With appropriate care, healthy older men and women do just as well with chemotherapy as younger individuals. Advances in supportive care (antinausea medicines and blood cell growth factors) have significantly decreased the side effects of chemotherapy and improved safety and the quality of life of older individuals with bladder cancer. Nonetheless, there is risk, especially if the patient is frail.

Because bladder cancer surgery can cause serious side effects and debilitation that requires significant healing time and energy, older patients usually tolerate neoadjuvant chemotherapy (given before surgery) better than adjuvant chemotherapy (given after surgery). On the other hand, because not all bladder cancer patients need chemotherapy (see Chapter 3), giving it after surgery (adjuvant therapy) offers the advantages of treating only those patients who absolutely need it. You should discuss the advantages and disadvantages of both approaches with your multi-disciplinary team.

With regard to choice of chemotherapy, healthy older patients can receive the same regimens as their younger counterparts, including those that are anthracycline-based, like MVAC (see Chapter 3). However, older patients are at increased risk of developing congestive heart failure from these regimens, and gemcitabine-cisplatin is probably a better choice, especially in those with a significant cardiac risk for anthracyclines. Recent studies have shown this regimen to be just as effective as MVAC but with fewer side effects.

Cisplatin is the cornerstone of all first-line chemotherapy regimens: neoadjuvant, adjuvant, and metastatic. However, this benefit is not without its downside. Older patients have a higher rate of severe side effects from cisplatin-based chemotherapy programs than those that use other drugs. This can be a major problem for those with kidney problems, congestive heart failure, or peripheral neuropathy from diabetes or other conditions that damage the nerves. Carboplatin is sometimes substituted for cisplatin in these patients. Taxane-based regimens are another alternative, but none of these alternate regimens has the same track record in fighting bladder cancer as those that contain cisplatin.

Managing chemotherapy-associated toxicity with appropriate supportive care is crucial in the elderly population to give them the best chance of cure and survival or to provide the best palliation. Reducing the dose of chemotherapy (or radiation therapy) based purely on chronological age may seriously affect the effectiveness of treatment. Those with metastatic disease may tolerate single-agent chemotherapy better, but the presence of severe comorbidities, age-related frailty, or underlying severe psychosocial problems may be obstacles, even for these treatment plans.

RADIATION THERAPY

As in younger patients, trimodal therapy with bladder preservation may be an option for selected older individuals with bladder cancer (see Chapter 3). It is an aggressive treatment approach that involves radiation therapy, chemotherapy, and surgery. If an older person is too frail to undergo radical cystectomy, he or she is usually too frail to get trimodal therapy. There are a few exceptions to this general rule, and it is essential that you weigh all of the risks and benefits with your multidisciplinary care team. In frail patients, radiation therapy is sometimes used to control the symptoms of bladder cancer, but it is rarely curative.

Radiation therapy usually provides excellent symptom relief (palliation) in metastatic and other incurable situations. It is also often quite effective in cancers that have recurred after initial surgery. It is particularly effective in treating pain caused by bladder cancer metastases to the bone. A short course of radiation therapy often allows patients with advanced cancer to lower (or even eliminate) their dose of narcotic pain relievers. Although these medicines do an excellent job of controlling pain, they often cause confusion, falls, and constipation in older patients. Thus even hospice patients suffering from localized metastatic bone pain should consider the option of palliative radiation therapy.

The fatigue that usually accompanies radiation therapy can be quite profound in the elderly, even in those who are fit. Often, the logistical details (like daily travel to the hospital for a 6-week course of treatment) are the hardest for older people. It is important that you discuss these potential problems with your family and social worker before starting radiation therapy.

COMMON TREATMENT COMPLICATIONS IN THE ELDERLY

Anemia (low red blood cell count) is common in the elderly, especially the frail elderly. It decreases the effectiveness of chemotherapy and often causes fatigue, falls, cognitive decline (for example, dementia, disorientation or confusion), and heart problems. Therefore it is essential that anemia be recognized and corrected with red blood cell transfusions or the appropriate use of erythropoiesis-stimulating agents like Procrit/Epogen (epoetin) or Aranesp (darbepoetin).

Myelosuppression (low white blood cell count) is also common in older patients getting chemotherapy or radiation therapy. Older patients with myelosuppression develop life-threatening infections more often than younger patients, and they may need to be treated in the hospital for many days. The liberal use of granulopoietic growth factors (G-CSF, Neupogen, Neulasta) decreases the risk of infection and makes it possible for older patients to receive full doses of potentially curable adjuvant chemotherapy.

Thrombocytopenia (low platelet cell count in the blood) can cause serious bleeding problems. This is especially worrisome in an older person who is prone to falling. Someone who bleeds into the brain can suffer a serious and debilitating stroke. Like anemia and myelosuppression, thrombocytopenia is a side effect of many chemotherapy medicines (especially carboplatin) and radiation therapy. It can usually be successfully managed by checking blood counts frequently and transfusing platelets when appropriate.

Mucositis (mouth sores) and diarrhea can cause severe dehydration in older patients who often are already dehydrated due to inadequate fluid intake and diuretics ("water pills" for high blood pressure or heart failure). Careful monitoring and the liberal use of antidiarrheal agents (Imodium) and oral and intravenous fluids are essential components of the management of older cancer patients, especially those receiving bladder radiation or 5-fluorouracil, or both.

Kidney function declines as we age. Some of the medicines that older patients take to treat both their cancer (for example, cisplatin, carboplatin, methotrexate, zoledronic acid, nonsteroidal anti-inflammatory drugs) and noncancer-related problems might make this worse. The dehydration that often accompanies cancer and its treatment can put additional stress on the kidneys. Fortunately, it is often possible to minimize these effects by carefully selecting and dosing appropriate drugs, managing "polypharmacy," and preventing dehydration.

Neurotoxicity and cognitive effects ("chemo-brain") can be profoundly debilitating in patients who are already cognitively impaired (demented, disoriented, confused, etc.). Elderly patients with a history of falling, hearing loss, or peripheral neuropathy (nerve damage from, for example, diabetes) have decreased energy and are highly vulnerable to neurotoxic chemotherapy like the taxanes or platinum compounds. Many of the medicines used to control nausea (antiemetics) or decrease the side effects of certain chemotherapeutic agents are also potential neurotoxins. These include dexamethasone (psychosis and agitation), ranitidine (agitation), diphenhydramine, and some of the antiemetics (sedation).

Fatigue is a near universal complaint of older cancer patients. It is particularly a problem for those who are socially isolated or depend on others to help them with activities of daily living. It is not necessarily related to depression, but it can be. Depression is quite common in the elderly. In contrast to younger patients who often respond to a cancer diagnosis with anxiety, depression is the more common disorder in older cancer patients. With proper support and medical attention, many of these patients can safely receive anticancer treatment.

Heart problems increase with age, and it is no surprise that older cancer patients have an increased risk of cardiac complications from intensive surgery, radiation, and chemotherapy. Because anthracyclines are known to increase the risk of congestive heart failure, the newer (neo) adjuvant chemotherapy regimens (gemcitabine/cisplatin) are better alternatives (to MVAC) for older men and women, especially those with a significant cardiac risk. Patients treated with cisplatin chemotherapy require large amounts of intravenous fluid hydration. This can cause congestive heart failure in patients with heart problems; they need careful monitoring.

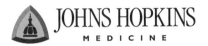

CHAPTER 11

JOHNS HOPKINS

MEDICINE

Trusted Resources—Finding Additional Information About Bladder Cancer and Its Treatment

Mark W. Ball

After receiving the diagnosis of cancer, many patients report that they hear very little else their doctor tells them. Although this information will be repeated and clarified over the ensuing visits with your physician, it can also be empowering to find out more information on your own. When searching for information about any healthcare topic, you should look for two criteria. First, the information should be published by a reliable source. Articles or reviews by experts are often the highest quality resources. Second, the information should be written at an appropriate level for the reader. Very technical writing may not be appropriate for everyone, whereas some patients may want more detailed scientific information. The following resources meet these criteria, are either expert written or reviewed, and offer varying levels of scientific detail.

BOOKS

The Guide to Living with Bladder Cancer is a very comprehensive yet easy to read book written by many experts in the field of bladder cancer. The original edition was written by Mark Schoenberg, MD, Professor of Urology and Oncology and the Faculty and Staff of the Johns Hopkins Genitourinary Oncology Group at the Johns Hopkins University School of Medicine. This book is an excellent resource and includes chapters on the anatomy of the urinary tract, overview of bladder cancer, symptoms, descriptions of surgical and nonsurgical options, as well as personal stories from bladder cancer patients.

100 Questions & Answer about Bladder Cancer, by Pamela Ellsworth, MD, and Brett Carswell, MD, is written in a question-and-answer style. At only 155 pages it is a quick read.

After Shock—What To Do When the Doctor Gives You—or Someone You Love—a Devastating Diagnosis, by Jessie Gruman, PhD, is a highly rated book that gives information on how to educate yourself about the disease, locate treatment options and specialists, obtain the best care, involve the support of family and friends, and handle career-related issues.

Bladder Cancer, Urostomy and Impotence, by Roni Olsen, wife of a bladder cancer patient, is available free to the public in pdf format at http://blcwebcafe.org/media/acrobat/bladder_cancer_urostomy_and_impotence.pdf

Bladder Cancer: A Resource Guide for Patients and Their Families, by Gary Dunetz, MD, a board-certified urologist, is a comprehensive yet easy-to-read guide aimed at improving dialogue with your physician.

Bladder Cancer: A Cleveland Clinic Guide, by Derek Raghavan, MD, and Kathleen Tuthill, is an illustrated guide that provides information for patients and loved ones with non-medical explanations.

ARTICLES

Articles from peer-reviewed medical journals offer quality information at a level for someone with some background in science. The following articles offer broad overviews about bladder cancer:

Amling, C. (2001). Diagnosis and management of superficial bladder cancer. *Current Problems in Cancer, 25*(4), 219–278.

Lee, R. L., & Droller, M. J. (2000). The natural history of bladder cancer: Implications for therapy. *Urologic Clinics of North America, 27*(1), 1–13.

van der Meijden, A. P. (1998). Fortnightly review: Bladder cancer. *BMJ, 317*(7169), 1366–1369.

Wai, C. Y., & Miller, D. S. (2002). Urinary bladder cancer. *Clinical Obstetrics and Gynecology, 45*(3), 844–854.

More articles about specific treatment options and the latest clinical trials may be accessed through the following resources:

Entrez-Pub Med

http://www.pubmed.gov

Pub Med is a search engine through the U.S. National Library of Medicine that includes over 18 million citations, biomedical articles including abstracts, links to full text articles, and related resources.

Medline Plus

http://www.nlm.nih.gov/medlineplus/
bladdercancer.html

Compilation of information about bladder cancer through the U.S. National Library of Medicine, including a list of current clinical trials and abstracts of the most up-to-date research.

ORGANIZATIONS

Many hospitals that treat bladder cancer have excellent sites devoted to the disease.

Brady Urological Institute

The Johns Hopkins Hospital
600 North Wolfe Street
Baltimore, MD 21287
410-955-6707
http://urology.jhu.edu/bladder

Includes information on basic anatomy, signs and symptoms, screening and diagnosis, treatment, resources, support services, information about patient care, and clinical trials taking place at Johns Hopkins.

Memorial Sloan-Kettering Cancer Center

1275 York Avenue
New York, NY 10065
212-639-2000
http://www.mskcc.org/mskcc/html/280.cfm

Includes information about symptoms, diagnosis, and treatment of bladder cancer and information about support groups and clinical trials taking place at Memorial Sloan-Kettering.

The University of Texas M. D. Anderson Cancer Center

1515 Holcombe Blvd.
Houston, TX 77030
1-800-392-1611
http://www.mdanderson.org/diseases/bladder

Includes an overview of bladder cancer, current news and articles, as well as information about clinical trials at M.D. Anderson.

United Ostomy Associations of America

http://www.uoaa.org
1-800-826-0826

National volunteer organization with over 200 chapters in the United States dedicated to assisting people who have had, will have, or are considering having intestinal or urinary diversions.

INTERNET RESOURCES

The Internet gives us access to a lot of information; however, it must be used with caution. Not all information is accurate or reviewed by experts—especially information from message boards or blogs.

The Bladder Cancer Web Café

http://blcwebcafe.org

An excellent starting point on the Web. It includes an overview of bladder cancer, treatment options, and survival guides written by patients. The content of the site is reviewed periodically for accuracy by an advisory board of experts in urologic oncology.

The Bladder Cancer Advocacy Network
http://www.bcan.org

Nonprofit organization of bladder cancer survivors, their families, and the medical community whose mission is to promote bladder cancer awareness. Its Web site is a wonderful resource that includes information for the newly diagnosed, information about current scientific research, and inspirational stories from survivors.

GENERAL INFORMATION

American Cancer Society
http://www.cancer.org
1-800-ACS-2345

Information about access to health care, statistics, research programs, and funding.

Cancer Survivors Network
http://csn.cancer.org

Includes discussion boards and chat rooms to meet and connect with other cancer survivors.

American Urological Association Foundation
http://www.urologyhealth.org

A site for patients written and reviewed by expert urologists in partnership with the American Urological Association Foundation.

National Cancer Institute
http://www.cancer.gov

Contains information about the Institute, including news, upcoming events, educational materials, and publications.

http://www.cancer.gov/cancertopics/types/bladder

National Cancer Institute's bladder cancer page includes an overview of the basics of bladder cancer.

SUPPORT SERVICES

Cancer Care
http://www.cancercare.org
1-800-813-HOPE

Includes information on telephone-based support groups.

Gilda's Club
http://www.gildasclub.org

Social and support community providing opportunities for networking and support groups as well as workshops, education, and social activities.

Lance Armstrong Foundation
http://www.livestrong.org

Information about support services, inspirational survivor stories, ways to get involved with fundraising and advocacy, grants, and community programs.

BCSisterhood
http://www.sylvialramsey.com/
bladdercancersisterhood.html

Blog and e-mail listserv created by survivor and advocate, Sylvia Ramsey, focusing on issues of special to concern women.

National Coalition for Cancer Survivorship

http://www.canceradvocacy.org

The oldest survivor-led advocacy organization in the country, devoted to bringing about change at the national level in how we research, finance, regulate, and deliver cancer care.

Patient Advocate Foundation

http://www.patientadvocate.org

Nonprofit organization that seeks to ensure financial stability, preservation of employment, and access to care for patients relative to their disease.

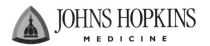

INFORMATION ABOUT
JOHNS HOPKINS

The James Buchanan Brady Urological Institute
(410) 955-6100: Appointment line
Author's email: mgonzalgo@gmail.com
http://www.urology.jhu.edu

The bladder cancer program at Johns Hopkins offers comprehensive, state-of-the-art bladder cancer diagnosis and treatment. A multi-disciplinary expert team consisting of surgeons, pathologists, radiation oncologists, and medical oncologists is available for consultation. The collaborative efforts of clinicians and researchers at the Brady Urological Institute have led to many advances in the treatment and understanding of the urinary tract and urinary tract cancer. The Web site features sections on diagnosis, treatment, drug development for noninvasive bladder cancer, pathology, clinical trials, and other valuable resource information.

About Johns Hopkins Medicine

Johns Hopkins Medicine unites physicians and scientists of the Johns Hopkins University School of Medicine with the organizations, health professionals, and facilities of the Johns Hopkins Health System. Its mission is to improve the health of the community and the world by setting the standard of excellence in medical education, research, and clinical care. Diverse and inclusive, Johns Hopkins Medicine has provided international leadership in the education of physicians and medical scientists in biomedical research and in the application of medical knowledge to sustain health since The Johns Hopkins Hospital opened in 1889.

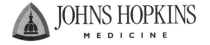

FURTHER READING

100 Questions & Answers About Overactive Bladder, Second Edition, Pamela Ellsworth & Alan J. Wein, Jones and Bartlett Publishers, 2010.

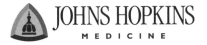

GLOSSARY

MARK W. BALL

Adjuvant therapy: Chemotherapy given shortly after surgery (before evidence of disease recurrence). This treatment is given in addition to surgery to prevent your cancer from coming back.

Anastomosis: Process through which two structures are joined or reconnected (i.e., a ureter to bowel anastomosis or bowel to urethra anastomosis).

Biopsy: Procedure that obtains tissue to analyze for cancer.

Bladder: Muscular organ that stores urine until it is time to void.

Cancer: Mutated cells that divide with uncontrolled growth potential.

Cell: The most basic unit of life that grows, reproduces, and contains genetic information in the form of DNA.

Chemotherapy: Drugs that kill rapidly dividing cancer cells; may also kill hair follicles and cells in the digestive system.

Continence: Ability to control bowel or bladder function.

CT: Imaging technique that uses x-rays and computers to construct slices of your body.

Cutaneous: Relating to or affecting the skin.

Cystoscopy: Technique in which a physician uses an instrument to view the inside of the urethra and bladder.

Electrocautery: A device that is used to stop bleeding with heat that is generated by an electric current.

Endoscopy: Visual examination of the inside of the body with the use of a fiberoptic scope.

Enterostomal nurse: Nurse specialized in the needs of patients with stomas.

Foley catheter: A flexible tube that is passed through the urethra into the bladder to drain urine.

Grade: Scale used by physicians that indicates how aggressive tumors appear under the microscope. The higher the number, the more aggressive the tumor.

Hematuria: Blood in the urine. Gross hematuria is seen with the naked eye, whereas microscopic hematuria is detected under the microscope.

Hospice: Specialized end-of-life care.

Ileal conduit: Reconstruction in which the ureters are implanted into part of the intestine called the ileum. This piece is brought to the skin, creating an opening called a stoma. Urine drains into a specialzed bag that is placed over the stoma.

Immunotherapy: Drugs that stimulate the body's own immune system to fight cancer cells.

Indiana pouch: An internal bladder traditionally made from large intestine (but can be made from small intestine) that is emptied by catheterizing. This type of urinary reconstruction may be created after radical cystectomy.

Intravenous pyelogram (IVP): Imaging technique that uses x-rays to visualized the kidneys, renal pelvis, and ureters.

Intravesical drug therapy: Chemotherapy delivered into the bladder.

Kidney: Paired organs that filter blood and make urine to be stored in the bladder.

Metastasis: Cancer that spreads to sites in the body distant to its origin.

Morbidity: The incidence of a disease or complication.

Mortality: The statistical calculation of death rates due to a specific disease within a population.

Multifocal tumors: Multiple tumors.

Neoadjuvant therapy: Chemotherapy given before surgery to decrease tumor size.

Oncology: Medical discipline that studies and treats cancer.

Orthotopic neobladder: A new bladder that is created from a piece of the intestine to permit voiding via the urethra.

Papillary: A type of tumor connected to the normal urothelium by a thin stalk.

Radiation oncology: Branch of medicine that uses radiation to treat cancer.

Radical cystectomy: Complete removal of the bladder and prostate (in a male) or removal of the bladder, uterus, and ovaries (in a female) for treatment of invasive bladder cancer.

Renal pelvis: Location within the kidney where urine is emptied. Urine is formed by the kidney and empties into the renal pelvis before traveling downstream into the ureter and then into the bladder where it is stored.

Sphincter: Round muscle that wraps around the base of the bladder and is important in maintaining continence.

Stage: System in which the size of a tumor, involvement of lymph nodes, and spread to distant sites in the body is used to calculate how advanced the cancer is. The higher the number, the more advanced the disease.

Stoma: An opening into the body from the outside created by a surgeon.

Stricture: Narrowing of a tube or connection (i.e., a urethral stricture or ureteral stricture).

Transitional epithelium: Layer of cells that line the renal pelvis, ureters, bladder, and urethra. Also known as urothelium.

Transurethral resection of bladder tumor (TURBT): Surgical removal of a bladder tumor through the urethra rather than through an open operation.

Tumor: A growth of cells. May either be benign or cancerous.

Ultrasound: Imaging technique that uses sounds waves to visualize structures.

Ureter: Tube that delivers urine from the kidney to the bladder where it is stored.

Urethra: Tube that delivers urine from the bladder to the outside of the body.

Urinalysis: Analysis of urine under a microscope to look for blood or evidence of infection.

Urothelium: Layer of cells that line the renal pelvis, ureters, bladder, and urethra. Also known as transitional epithelium.

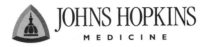

INDEX